DATE DUE

CLASSIFI

PRACTI

GAYLORD   PRINTED IN U.S.A.

LANGUAGES AND LINGUISTICS

Additional books in this series can be found on Nova's website
under the Series tab.

Additional E-books in this series can be found on Nova's website
under the E-book tab.

NEUROLOGY - LABORATORY AND CLINICAL RESEARCH DEVELOPMENTS

Additional books in this series can be found on Nova's website
under the Series tab.

Additional E-books in this series can be found on Nova's website
under the E-book tab.

APHASIA

CLASSIFICATION, MANAGEMENT PRACTICES AND PROGNOSIS

EDVIN HOLMGREN

AND

ELLINOR S. RUDKILDE

EDITORS

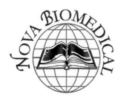

New York

LIBRARY OF CONGRESS CATALOGING-IN-PUBLICATION DATA

Aphasia : classification, management practices, and prognosis / editors, Edvin Holmgren and Ellinor S. Rudkilde.
       p. cm.
 Includes bibliographical references and index.
 ISBN 978-1-62257-681-4
 1. Aphasia. I. Holmgren, Edvin. II. Rudkilde, Ellinor S.
 RC425.A634 2013
 616.85'5206--dc23

Published by Nova Science Publishers, Inc. † New York

Contents

Preface

Aphasia is an acquired impairment of production or comprehension of language or both resulting from damage to the language network in the brain. In this book, the authors present topical research in the study of the classification, management practices and prognosis of an aphasia diagnosis. Topics discussed include aphasia consequences to the patient and care-givers; the clinical patterns of aphasia; intensive treatment, pharmacotherapy, transcranial magnetic/electric stimulation as a potential adjuvant treatment for aphasia; diagnosis and management of language impairment in acute stroke; and aphasia classifications.

Chapter I - This chapter describes consequences from aphasia from the perspective of those affected and their close relatives. Nine persons with lived experiences of aphasia contribute to data by means of interviews, published books and diaries, and seventeen close relatives narrated about their situation as informal caregivers. All that information was interpreted in three parts in accordance with a lifeworld hermeneutic approach. The first, which dealt with existential consequences of aphasia, indicated that the intentional, non-verbal act when something is recognized *as* something is *not* affected by aphasia. Aphasia merely affects the world of symbols, which is necessary for interaction with others. It is therefore connected with feelings of alienation, inferiority and shame in social settings. The second part, which dealt with the issue of professional aphasia care, suggests that adequate care from the affected person's point of view presupposes a secure base and a caregiver who recognizes and trusts the patient's ability to think and communicate albeit not always verbally. In the third part the investigation is directed to close relative's situation. It is suggested that a life together with an aphasic person means being used as a bridge between the aphasic person and the surrounding world.

This leaves close relatives with a lonely burden of responsibility. Finally a synthesizing analyse suggests that aphasia management practice includes care and support as a mutual concern and a shared responsibility for professional carers, close relatives and community service. The principles for that are outlined under seven main heads.

Chapter II - From the simplistic explanations of Wernicke's and Broca's, to the latest investigative headways made into the understanding of intricacies involved in the use of the spoken and written words; modern science is still in the process of understanding Aphasias. The use of radiological and pathological diagnostic modalities in the study of language deficits has helped in the recognition of two categories of aphasias. The acute and sub-acute presentations seen mostly in association with cerebrovascular accidents, CNS infections, and head trauma shows involvement of specific parts of the perisylvian language network which is located in the left hemisphere in majority of right as well as left-handed individuals. Based upon the evaluation of spontaneous speech, naming, comprehension, repetition, reading and writing, and diagnostic imaging these aphasias are divided into central aphasias and the disconnection syndromes. The central aphasias, namely Wernicke's and Broca's are due to damage of the two classical, though not anatomically discrete language centers bearing the same names. The disconnection syndromes are a result of damage to areas of the language network other than the classical centers and include Transcortical and Conduction Aphasias among others. The slowly progressive aphasias caused by neurodegenerative diseases are referred to as Primary progressive aphasias (PPA). In order to simplify understanding of these aphasias and thereby help find cures these aphasias have recently been classified into the agrammatic, semantic, and logopenic variants. Management and prognostic issues pertaining exclusively to language disruption are widely studied in the aphasias with actual presentation. The mainstay of treatment is speech and language therapy; however some drugs are also showing promise especially when combined with language therapy. In post-stroke aphasic patients there is a strong correlation between initial severity and eventual recovery. Although most improvement occurs in the first few months, late language therapy has also shown benefit. Ongoing research also points to the potential utility of transcranial magnetic and electric stimulation for the treatment of certain aphasias.

Chapter III - Aphasia after stroke is a common and disabling symptom, which can recover in the weeks, months or years following brain injury, showing that the adult brain can reorganize to adjust to impaired functions.

Standard rehabilitation approaches aim to improve the deficient function through speech and language therapy (SLT). In parallel with increasing knowledge about central nervous system plasticity, different adjuvant interventions have been recently implemented to enhance the outcome of speech and language therapy. One of them consists in increasing the intensity of SLT in order to obtain better recovery. This is achieved for instance with computer-assisted therapy (CAT) or with constraint-induced aphasia therapy (CIAT) approaches.

A second approach tested the combination of a number of drugs with SLT, with the aim to increase its effect. The mechanism thought to underlie enhanced recovery with the addition of specific drugs includes increasing attention and learning though modulation of neurotransmission or restoring metabolic function. Several substances have been assessed, including noradrenergic drugs and drugs acting on the dopaminergic, glutaminergic, gabaergic, and cholinergic systems.

Finally, another, still experimental, intervention in stroke rehabilitation consists of neuromodulation via non-invasive cortical stimulation, e.g. through transcranial magnetic stimulation (TMS) or direct current stimulation (tDCS). These techniques have recently been proposed to potentially endorse functional recovery after stroke through (i) enhancing excitability of the stroke hemisphere or (ii) suppressing the non-stroke hemisphere to reduce its potential interference with functional recovery of the stroke hemisphere.

While both treatment intensity and TMS have led to several promising results on efficacy in aphasia rehabilitation, the effect of pharmacotherapy seems to be less straightforward. In the present chapter we will perform a review of recent literature on the effects of these approaches as potential adjuvant to standard SLT in the rehabilitation of aphasia.

Chapter IV - Language impairments are frequent in stroke, especially in the hyper acute phase, occurring in 15 to 50% of stroke patients. Recovery from aphasia remains difficult to predict. Language impairment still exists in at least 50% of initially aphasic patients one year after stroke. Post-stroke aphasia is a major source of disability that can lead to impaired communication, reduced social activities, depression and a decreased likelihood of resuming work. The role of the stroke unit in improving morbidity, mortality and recovery has been clearly demonstrated. Nevertheless, the need for intense and sustained acute management of aphasia in specialized stroke units remains controversial. The recent validation of a tool to rapidly screen for aphasia (LAST) after stroke allows for its early detection and management. Early detection of aphasia after stroke may improve outcomes by taking advantage of the synergy between intensive speech therapy and early neural reorganization. Daily re-evaluation will facilitate tailored rehabilitation sessions, multidisciplinary management by the stroke team, and development of educational resources for patients and their caregivers. Standardizing protocols for identifying and managing aphasia requires the co-operation and coordination of the entire stroke team, along with the daily presence of speech therapists. These considerations are crucial for patients in the stroke unit to achieve the full benefit of the management proposed in this chapter, to ultimately promote better long term functional prognosis.

Chapter V - In this chapter it is emphasized that there are only two fundamental forms of aphasia, which are linked to impairments in the lexical/semantic and grammatical systems of language (Wernicke-type aphasia and Broca-type aphasia, respectively). Other aphasic syndromes do not really impair language knowledge per se, but rather either some peripheral mechanisms required to produce language (conduction aphasia and aphasia of the supplementary motor area), or the executive control of the language (extra-Sylvian or transcortical motor aphasia). A new classification of aphasic syndromes is suggested. In this proposed classification a distinction is established between primary (or ''central'') aphasias (Wernicke's aphasia—three subtypes—and Broca's aphasia); secondary (or ''peripheral'') aphasias (conduction aphasia and supplementary motor area aphasia); and dysexecutive aphasia.

In: Aphasia   ISBN: 978-1-62257-681-4
Editors: E. Holmgren, E.S. Rudkilde   © 2013 Nova Science Publishers, Inc.

Chapter I

Aphasia Management Practice: Care and Support – A Mutual Concern and a Shared Responsibility

Maria Nyström
Borås University, School of Health Sciences, Borås, Sweden

Abstract

This chapter describes consequences from aphasia from the perspective of those affected and their close relatives. Nine persons with lived experiences of aphasia contribute to data by means of interviews, published books and diaries, and seventeen close relatives narrated about their situation as informal caregivers. All that information was interpreted in three parts in accordance with a lifeworld hermeneutic approach. The first, which dealt with existential consequences of aphasia, indicated that the intentional, non-verbal act when something is recognized *as* something is *not* affected by aphasia. Aphasia merely affects the world of symbols, which is necessary for interaction with others. It is therefore connected with feelings of alienation, inferiority and shame in social settings. The second part, which dealt with the issue of professional aphasia care, suggests that adequate care from the affected person's point of view presupposes a secure base and a caregiver who recognizes and trusts the patient's ability to think and communicate albeit not always verbally. In the third part the investigation is directed to close relative's situation. It is suggested that a life together with an aphasic person means being used as a bridge between the aphasic person and the surrounding world. This leaves close relatives with a lonely burden of responsibility. Finally a synthesizing analyse suggests that aphasia management practice includes care and support as a mutual concern and a shared responsibility for professional carers, close relatives and community service. The principles for that are outlined under seven main heads.

Introduction

Many models for recovery from aphasia processes do not take into account that remaining speech impairments lead to difficulties in interacting with friends and relatives, which in turn, can delay recovery. This chapter on aphasia management practice therefore concentrates on interpersonal relations as a secure base for further rehabilitation.

Aphasia victims meet professional carers from the on-set of their illness. Yet in a literature review Tacke (1999) found no research investigating the carer's significance for the results of the aphasia treatment. On the contrary the review shows that carers working in general hospitals rarely centred their attention on the individual needs of the aphasic patient, with the result that there is little interaction between carers and patients during the hospital stay.

However, interest in caring science research has increased during the 21st century, and it has been found that professional carers can provide support that enhances the patient's self-esteem and help them to gain a positive but realistic view of the situation. Adequate caring might even encourage progress towards rehabilitation, and turn a blocked situation into a secure one. Andersson and Fridlund (2002) found that interactions with professionals were adequate when they balanced and compensated for disabilities. Sundin and Janson (2003) observed patient-carer interactions during morning care, and they interviewed excellent carers, who were recommended for the study by colleagues. Those professional carers neither reflected nor talked much during caring; instead they used their hands to communicate through touching. The carers thought that talking disturbed the ability of severely aphasic patients' to concentrate.

Caring measures also need to take existential issues that follow on from aphasia into account. That is particularly important preventing the development of post-stroke depression. Depression is a common experience related to coping with post-stroke effects and has a negative impact on rehabilitation (Robinson, 2002). Depressed persons with aphasia often suffer from reduced self-esteem, which may change their self-image Depression may further affect the motivation needed to improve functional independence, as failure to participate in the community due to impaired verbal ability often results in feelings of loneliness and isolation.

That the effectiveness of conventional therapies has not been conclusively proven (c.f. Berthier, 2005) has led to attempts to integrate knowledge from several therapeutic domains in efforts to introduce other strategies. Cunningham (1998) suggested a counselling approach for patients with severe aphasia, in order to facilitate adaptation to the situation. Van der Gaag et al. (2005) proposed that therapeutic approaches should include family members in order to improve quality of life and communication, as most caregiving is provided by close relatives, at least in the long run.

Research into informal caregiving also emphasizes the importance of non-professional careproviders (Lau and McKenna, 2001). Yet little research is directed to close relatives' problems in an abruptly changed life situation (c.f. Sawatzky and Fowler-Kerry, 2003; Blake, Lincoln and Clark, 2003; Tooth et.al 2005). The same is true for close relatives' educational needs (c.f. O'Connell and Baker, 2003).

According to Bäckström and Sundin (2007) close relatives of stroke survivors often sacrifice themselves and disregard their own needs. Wallengren, Friberg and Segesten (2008) describe such experiences as being "shadows", partly because they are invisible to professional caregivers who focus entirely on the patients and frequently forget their families.

The ability and willingness of close relatives to understand and respond to the aphasic person seems nevertheless to be of vital importance. This is in clear contrast to the amount of attention that has been paid to specific problems from the perspective of informal caregivers.

The starting point for the study that now follows is the assumption that we need knowledge about the consequences of aphasia as an existential challenge in order to provide adequate care and support, which in turn can serve as a firm base for further rehabilitation. The first part describes the experience of suffering stroke and aphasia and the struggle to regain the ability to communicate. The second part describes the conditions needed for properly functioning professional aphasia care, seen from aphasic persons' viewpoint. The third part concerns those closely related to an aphasic person, and their need for support from community service.[1] Finally the three parts are

---

[1] The three parts were initially interpreted separately and have been published as three different papers (Nyström 2006; 2009; 2011).

compared and synthesized in order to reach a further understanding on how to provide a firm and solid caring base for a person with aphasia, which can serve as a foundation for further rehabilitation.

Study Design - A Lifeworld Hermeneutic Approach

The study has a lifeworld hermeneutic design. Lifeworld research emphasizes individuals as living wholes and focuses on the world as it is experienced prior to the formulating of any hypothesis to explain it (Dahlberg, Dahlberg and Nyström, 2008). It does not look at objects and events as such, but at the way in which they are perceived and experienced as phenomena. Lifeworld research basically draws on the works of the philosophers Edmund Husserl (1970) and Hans-George Gadamer (1997).

The interpretative analysis was inspired by Paul Ricoeur (1976). It was through the dialectic of understanding or explanation that Ricoeur developed his interpretation theory, in which understanding and explanation overlap and cross each other. The range of propositions and meanings in the set of data, which is described below, has thus been unfolded in the phases of explanation.

Understanding emerges from the chain of partial meanings moving toward a whole in an act of synthesis, and it relies on the meaningfulness of expressions such as vocal and written signs. This is in accordance with Ricoeur who suggested that understanding, explanation, and interpretation are mutual forms of the concept of understanding that rely on the same sphere of meaning.

In approaching the issues involved in suffering from aphasia, professional aphasia care and being closely related to an aphasic person, interpretations necessarily involve several attempts to explain meanings in the data. For this reason, theories from existential philosophy and psychodynamics are sometimes used as analytical tools. When that is the case the theoretic tool is briefly mentioned in the findings.

Four women and five men, aged 45-72 at the time of data collection, participated in the first two parts of the study. The data comprise transcribed interviews, autobiographies and excerpts from diaries. Data were collected in Sweden, from nine Swedish-speaking informants, who made their contributions to the data set on 16 different occasions. They were purposefully selected from among members of two branches of the Swedish National

Fellowship for Aphasia, in order to obtain variation in age, gender, type of aphasia and timelapse since occurrence of the cerebral lesion. Type of aphasia was reported by the informants themselves or their spouses.

During the interviews it was necessary to communicate in a way that facilitated understanding. Some interviewees could speak adequately, while others still exhibited the symptoms of expressive and/or impressive aphasia. One important criterion, which limited the number of potential interviewees, was the need to communicate relatively well, orally and/or in writing. In this study communication includes both explicit and implicit meanings that are expressed and interpreted in social intercourse. The interviewees had thus either recovered or learned how to carry on a conversation in spite of the difficulties of speaking or understanding words.

The interviews followed the principles of the life-world approach mentioned above. The interviewees were invited to reflect as openly and deeply as possible on their experiences of aphasia, their struggle to regain the ability to communicate, and their experiences of aphasia care. These interviews were audio-taped and transcribed verbatim.

When more information was required in order to establish the relevance of a tentative interpretation, some informants were contacted again for follow-up interviews. In these interviews the questions were more specific and aimed at obtaining information that could further illuminate the relevance of tentative interpretations (see validity criteria below). The follow-up interviews were not audio-taped but notes were made.

Three interviewees supplemented their interviews with written material that further illuminated their statements. These included diaries or written advice from the interviewees to others with aphasia. Two autobiographies that described experiences of aphasia (Tropp-Erblad, 2002/1882; Dahlin, 1997) were also used as data, but were complemented with interviews. Time lapse since the occurrence of the brain lesion varied from 1-23 years.

The close relatives, 11 women and 6 men, who were interviewed for the third part of the study were purposefully chosen through the aphasia associations. As it was presumed there would be variations in community service they were selected from three different Swedish municipalities, a big city, a smaller town and a rural municipality.

There were 10 spouses, 6 adult children and one parent of aphasic persons. These interviews also followed the principles of an open life-world approach, and all began with a question about what it is like to be closely related to a person with aphasia. The interviewees were encouraged to describe their experiences and their actual life situation as deeply as possible. Pliable probing questions were asked in order to get them to reflect on matters that were not at first described.

Interpretative Analysis

Within the three texts statements were compared and put together according to similarities so that further meanings could be abstracted from the data. Tentative interpretations emerged, each illuminating one aspect of the complexity that characterized personal experiences of aphasia, professional care and the situation as close relative. The relevance of the tentative interpretations was evaluated using the following validity criteria:

- The source of an interpretation should only be an actual piece of the data. If theoretical support is used, it is merely as a tool to suggest explanations for a certain item of information. Thus no theory must guide the whole interpretative process.
- No other interpretations should be found that better (more meaningfully) explain the same data.
- There must be no contradictions between an interpretation and the data.
- When more information is required in order to establish the relevance of a tentative interpretation, informants must be contacted again for follow-up interviews.

All interpretations that were deemed to be valid were compared with each other in order to arrive at a comprehensive understanding for each analytical part of the study. In the final synthetizing analysis all three parts were compared, with the following validity criteria in mind:

- The level of abstraction is connected to the principle of moving from the parts to the whole and vice versa, striving for consistency in the jigsaw puzzle of interpretation.
- The consistency of the picture that emerges must be further strengthened by ensuring that no data of general importance are omitted from the synthetizing analysis.

The First Analysis

Existential Consequences of Aphasia

The following first interpretative analysis is based on data from nine informants with personal experiences of suffering a stroke with aphasia. They are also familiar with the struggle to regain the capacity to communicate. As mentioned above, they contributed to the data in several ways by means of interviews, auto biographies and diaries.

Below six interpretations are presented of that information which covers six different aspects of the research phenomenon; existential consequences of aphasia. A comparison of these different aspects culminates in a comprehensive understanding that illuminates the existential meaning of losing the world of symbols. The quotations are excerpted from the data.

It is Essential to Repress Feelings in Order to Act Rationally During the Acute Phase

Despite the fact that warning signs, such as TIA or venal thrombosis, were common, all the interviewees experienced their aphasia as a bolt from the blue. For some, all verbal communication suddenly ceased; while others could speak fluently but without making any sense. Finding oneself in such a situation was generally perceived as a horrific experience, although in retrospect it was only partly associated with feelings of shock and fear.

When the stroke occurred only one interviewee became unconscious, while the others were confused and unable to act rationally. One of them recalled that she just wanted to take a nap and lie down in the snow beside her car. For another, the first indication of a brain lesion was somewhat unusual; he bid on everything at an auction. Those who were less confused recognized that they must act in order to get help, and afterwards they were surprised by their ability to act rationally. One man, for example, was alone in his weekend cottage when it happened and knew immediately that he was unfit to drive. He understood that he had to walk quite a distance in order to contact his neighbour.

Some concluded that the capacity to repress feelings of shock and fear is due to a biological process associated with their cerebral lesion, while others explained their calmness as a mix of biological and psychological processes.

> Your body cannot accept that you cannot speak. You can't understand it emotionally. (Is this, do you think, due to the cerebral lesion?) No, not just the lesion, it is also a psychological process.

Such statements indicate that the calm is experienced as a process of repressing feelings as a result of psychological defence mechanisms, such as isolation and rationalisation. The concept of isolation is used by ego psychologists (Freud, 1966; Blanck and Blanck, 1974) to describe mental processes where feelings are separated from thoughts. Isolation as a personal characteristic can indeed be problematic, but it is also an important resource in moments of threat and panic. The isolation of feelings seems in fact to make it possible to put thoughts aside in order to act in a rational manner. The man who became aware of his aphasia while alone in his weekend cottage knew immediately that he must repress his feelings in order to get help and employed his isolation and rationalisation skills as a conscious strategy, contrary to the theory of psychological defence-mechanisms, as an unconscious phenomenon.

> When I recognised that I could neither speak nor write I understood immediately that it was important to remain calm and take one thing at time, and I repeated that to myself every time I was almost seized by panic.

After arrival at the hospital it was possible to stop repressing feelings. This supports the interpretation that feelings are repressed only when it is essential to act rationally. On the other hand, other interviewees stayed calm for a long time, even after their arrival at the hospital. One woman was unaffected by her severe communication disabilities for a period of two years. It was not until she started to speak again that she became frustrated and angry when she was unable to communicate.

It thus appears impossible to fully explain the calmness in the acute phase of aphasia. Nevertheless, it seems fair to conclude that it is important to be able to repress feelings in an acute situation when it is urgent that decisions are made about how to get help.

Emotional Life Is Intertwined with the Struggle to Regain Language

Some interviewees regained the power of speech within three months, but others still exhibited greater or lesser impediments of language, both oral and written, at the time of the data collection. They spoke slowly and now and then failed to find the right words. Some also found it difficult to understand non-verbal expressions, such as nodding for yes and shaking the head to indicate no.

Others could neither count nor estimate time. One woman could not read or write, while others had difficulties writing. A few interviewees failed to understand some questions during the interview, mostly abstract ones. In such cases, being allowed to read the questions increased their ability to communicate.

As time passed and their ability to communicate improved, the interviewees successively became increasingly frustrated and angry at their failure to express their thoughts and/or understand what other people were saying.

> Nowadays I am so angry about not being able to speak properly. It [the ability to speak] can be locked away when something else, such as a headache, is bothering me. It is so infernally hard and arduous to think and speak.

One woman recalled two mute years and described a sense of tranquillity that afterwards became totally inadequate for her. When she was unable to express herself she had a feeling of being on the point of death, where nothing seemed to really matter. Another woman said that her head was emptied of all thoughts during the period of severe aphasia.

> It was so odd, as if there was no activity in the brain. It must have been the stroke and the oedema in the brain.

After a period of successful speech training, this woman became anxious and frightened, as she felt pressurised by the idea that if one failed to regain the power of speech within five years one would remain mute forever. Other interviewees also reported that their calmness disappeared when they began to speak again, thus implying thatthe force driving them to speak increased in line with their anxiety. One interviewee, who had recovered from impressive aphasia, recalled having many words in her head but that they were just a chaotic mess. Initially she was calm, because she was able to understand and believed the physicians' reassurances that she would recover. Feelings of anxiety, fear and anger seemed, however, to increase in line with her successful efforts to regain the use of language.

For one interviewee, the acute phase of aphasia coincided with the death of her son. She could not cry "properly", her body just shook. Furthermore, she could not stand being close to others, not even her own family. When she regained her speech she started to cry and work through the sorrow in her heart and was pleased to have her family by her side.

Is language a precondition for feelings and feelings a precondition for language? If so, it would be impossible to explain sadness, rage and anxiety among infants and animals. It seems more reasonable to assume that increased activity and capacity in the brain trigger feelings of despair, and the struggle to regain the power of speech as well as the ability to communicate. Such experiences are probably best understood as an interwoven process of biological and existential conditions that enable the most significant of human abilities: language. Thus it appears important that the initial calmness disappears in order to make room for a fighting spirit.

It Is Not Necessary to Name the World in Order to Recognize Its Meaning

Some psychologists (cf. Blanck and Blanck, 1974) emphasize verbal language as a precondition for thought, especially those thoughts that are necessary for formal operations. In the present study the interviewees with expressive aphasia were silent, even inside their heads, but were by no means devoid of thoughts. They claimed to have been able to grasp meaning without access to words. One of them described how "words ran out of my head" with amazement and confusion. He found that in spite of the total silence inside his head he could still think, albeit non-verbally.

> It is not true that you cannot think without words. I just stood there and analyzed the situation. I was totally calm, incomprehensibly tranquil as a matter of fact, and I discovered another language, a nonverbal language, and it worked!

This interviewee talked about a "meta-language", a non-verbal and silent language, which, according to him, may be hidden behind the verbal language and therefore inaccessible to a person who can speak. He stated that this "meta-language" is complete in itself and consists of entireties, whole meanings. These meanings are experienced as absolute truth, you do not consider any other options or alternatives as meaning already exists.

All interviewees, despite their different types of aphasia, claimed that they had been aware of everything around them in their waking life, despite the fact that they could not communicate anything about it to other people.

> I can't explain exactly how it was. I knew that I could think, and I did think, but I don't recall any words.

One interviewee, who was unconscious after the stroke, found that she was mute when she regained consciousness. When she tried to shake her head for no and nod to indicate yes everything went wrong. Her head was empty; she had no access to any words with which to communicate. After a while she recognized single words from time to time, but no coherent language.

Nevertheless, she claimed that she understood everything that was going on around her. Another interviewee knew immediately that he must act in order to get help. He could neither speak nor write, but he could consider his options and ponder alternatives, so as to obtain assistance. A third individual, who had experience of impressive aphasia, claimed to have been able to understand concrete as well as abstract matters in spite of the chaotic language inside his head.

A few interviewees appeared, however, not to understand all the questions during the interview. One of them said that he had learned to maintain the initiative in a conversation in order to avoid situations that included interpretations of another person's verbal messages. When given time during the interview he proved capable of adequately answering questions that were concrete and complemented by gestures and/or written words. He related that, after four years with impressive aphasia, he had learned how to get a rough understanding.

We may all have experience of word-less and holistic meanings in our dreams, and it seems reasonable to interpret the "meta-language" described by one interviewee and the immediate understanding described by most of the others, as an un-reflected dreamlike recognition that does not require words.

In common withsome of the interviewees in this study, we are not always as upset as we might have reason to be during the surrealistic experience of dreaming. When we wake up we can be overwhelmed by feelings, but cannot understand the feelings without reflection. Reflection requires access to words. Interpretation of dreams also presupposes language (Freud, 1968). Similarly some interviewees in this study reflected on their initial dreamlike condition for the first time during the research interview.

Worrying About Being Considered Stupid

Becoming fully aware of the consequences of aphasia appears to be both frightening and humiliating, despite regaining the ability to communicate. One man, who had regained all his communication skills at the time of the data collection, recalled his awareness of the gravity of his condition when a physician talked to him to give him an overall picture of his brain lesion, without saying anything about rehabilitation.

> It was a shock! The physician pointed to the wall and asked me what
> it was. The words were not there, I couldn't name anything. Nothing was
> there!

Another interviewee, who immediately understood his disastrous
situation, described in his diary feelings of rage, humiliation and despair, when
he realized after some time that his communication impairment would remain,
even when the physical consequences of the stroke had more or less abated.

> To just sit there mute and stupid, with one's head full of more or less
> brilliant comments, not being able to make use of them, it is trying,
> dreadfully trying, and it makes me very angry. I feel totally worthless,
> like a parcel labelled: "worthless sample".

Several interviewees were in the habit of always using bank notes when
they went shopping, in order to avoid the humiliation of failing to hand over
the right coins to the salesperson. A communication impediment, or worse,
total muteness, was thus experienced as a much more devastating individual
catastrophe than any physical handicap. The interviewees described feelings of
being locked inside their bodies. They lost their sense of dignity because they
were unable to communicate adequately. Verbal language was experienced as
a prerequisite for participating in society, and without language they thought
that they were considered stupid. The interviewees' self-esteem and sense of
dignity were thus threatened by their own interpretations of other people's
assessments of their capacity to think and talk properly.

> When I lost my speech I lost my sense of security. As I had no
> words, I couldn't give expression to nuances. When I could not speak I
> appeared to be a person who could not think in shades of meaning. It was
> impossible for me to change that, I simply had to put up with other
> people's way of looking at me.

Existential Loneliness Causes Feelings of Alienation

Most interviewees also claimed that the healthcare system abandoned
them, because no professional caregiver supported them in their early efforts
to regain the power of speech. Some of them started to practise words at night
in the hospital, soon after the onset of their condition, in spite of
recommendations to rest and take it easy. A librarian, as opposed to a care-
provider, understood one man's mute plea for something to read, after which
he started to recall words. In another case, it was the patient's 12-year-old

grandson who wrote words on flash cards, to be used for communicating care needs. The absence of professional support in the interviewees' struggle to regain speech gave rise to feelings of loneliness, but even more devastating were the serious consequences for their private interpersonal relations.

> If everything previously well-known appears strange, and communication with those around you is cut off, then the soul is incarcerated in an impenetrable prison, it must be the loneliest soul in the world.

A previously unknown feeling of loneliness, which increases and extends to all domains of everyday life, can thus follow the single-handed struggle to regain the ability to communicate.

Feelings of being alone, imprisoned in the body, appear to create a distance to other people. Some of the interviewees no longer knew who they were, because of their inability to communicate adequately. Their identity seemed to vanish and they considered themselves merely as handicapped people. Not knowing who you are and being unable to maintain your self-esteem makes it easy to distrust the good intentions of others.

> When B called he said that my speech was much better than last time he talked to me. But last time he said that I spoke just as well as before the stroke.

Existential loneliness seems to increase when other people ignore or make light of the communication impairments. In the most harrowing moments there are feelings of alienation that include both internal life and the surrounding world. One woman, who used to enjoy her own company when thinking and talking to herself, found that she was not the same person inside when she suffered from impressive aphasia. It made her feel completely alone. In the following statement she describes her feelings of alienation after being unsuccessful at an evening course in English.

> The last bus was very crowded. I looked at the people. It was like a Brecht play, as if they were wearing masks. I could not see the faces behind the masks, and their eyes were like empty hollows. I got off the bus and started to walk home. When I arrived home my husband looked at me. He was also wearing a mask!

Strategies for Handling Communication Problems Help to Create Some Distance to the Situation

Many statements could be interpreted as strategies for regaining control over a life situation, despite an impaired ability to communicate. As described above, the strategy aimed at regaining control could start with an immediate and single-handed fight to learn to speak again with no help from professional caregivers, who were considered negligent in terms of their responsibility to assist patients in this struggle.

For others, who continued to suffer from the effects of impressive aphasia, it remained difficult to interpret messages from other people. One strategy that could reduce the instances of humiliation was to control any conversation by choosing the topic, which increased the chances of guessing the meaning of the talk. This strategy, however, was not always successful because of the risk of being excluded from the conversation if one guessed incorrectly. Under such circumstances, giving up could be the easiest way out. A more successful strategy was to ask other people to speak slowly, in order to increase the time available for understanding a verbal message. This may be a similar strategy to the one previously mentioned, i.e. avoiding paying with small change.

Other activities that could be interpreted as strategies for increasing control, especially among those who had been successfully rehabilitated, were commitment to other persons with aphasia, either professionally or in non-profit making organisations. Yet another was not to be afraid to make a fool of oneself.

Friends who failed to recognize them as the same person as before the stroke were not considered real friends. Another way to control the situation was to maintain one's self-esteem and dignity with the help of humour and self-irony. Using humour in such a way may serve as an internal triumph in a life situation that might otherwise be hard to manage.

> Sometimes I made fun of myself just to make things easier. But I was deeply concerned and frightened.

A common denominator among the different strategies was that they created a distance between oneself and one's problems and motivated the interviewees to undertake various measures. Involvement in something other than problems, also appeared to increase well-being, *for* example taking an interest in the resources available for rehabilitation and policies for prioritising healthcare problems.

To Lose the World of Symbols - Comprehensive Understanding

When the nine persons who described their experiences of aphasia fell ill they were unconscious, confused, or wide-awake and recording what was happening. In spite of initial shock and fear, the following period of silence or unconnected, inadequate words in the head was like a dreamlike state characterized by a surrealistic sense of total calm in the eye of a storm. The external world was experienced as an unconditional entity that could be grasped without being able to talk, and sometimes not even understand, what others were saying. The phenomenological theory of intentionality may help in understanding such a non-verbal, pre-reflective grasp of reality. In employing the concept of "intentionality", Husserl had no doubt about the inherent power of what he called the "natural attitude", i.e. "the everyday immersion in one's existence and experience, in which we take for granted that the world is as we perceive it, and that others experience the world as we do"(Husserl, 1970 in Dahlberg et al. 2008). In the act of intentionality we do not critically reflect, we are merely in the everyday world in which we live.

When the interviewees in this study were stricken with aphasia, they appeared to lose the ability to move from intentional consciousness to reflection. The world around them was taken for granted in the same way as the air they breathed. They obviously did not find it necessary to analyse their experiences, but appeared to remain in intentionality during the time that they had no access to words.

Is it possible to intentionally recognize reality without words? According to Merleau-Ponty (1989), one of Husserl's followers, such a conclusion seems eminently reasonable. Words are not a precondition for thought. On the contrary, thought is a precondition for language.

> It [the word] is not without meaning, since behind it there is a categorical operation, but this meaning is something which it does not have, does not possess, since it is thought which has a meaning, the word remaining an empty container. It is merely a phenomenon of articulation, of sound, or the consciousness of such phenomenon, but in any case language is but an external accompaniment of thought (Merleau-Ponty, 1989 p.177).

A further aspect of intentionality is the ability to think in entireties, without words, immediately after being struck by aphasia. Most of the interviewees not only grasped and recognised their reality, but were later surprised at their own calmness as well as their ability to cope with the acute situation. Even those with strong elements of impressive aphasia remembered and were able to describe the acute phase, despite the fact that they were confused when it occurred.

Hence, aphasia reduces neither perception nor the immediate ability to recognise something *as* something, rather the reverse. The act of intentionality appears to be a more powerful experience than ever before when words are lost; it was interpreted as a "meta-language" by one interviewee in the study.

Instead, the devastating consequence of aphasia is its effect on interpersonal life, one's ability to interact with others. Interaction presupposes symbols and signs that mean something in accordance with convention within a specific cultural context (Charon, 1989). Words, money, signs and many non-verbal expressions of meaning are examples of symbols. In order to communicate we must make use of significant symbols that are accepted as carriers of meaning in our society. Communication also involves the ability to generate a certain meaning in the minds of others, as well as the capacity to understand what others want to say. Impaired symbolization capacity was exemplified in this study by the interviewees' difficulty in using coins, estimating time and understanding gestures and so on. Most devastating of all was, of course, the loss of those symbols that are important for language. It was not just the written or spoken word itself that appeared to be devoid of meaning but also complementary symbols associated with speech, such as nodding for yes and shaking one's head to indicate no, recognizing expressions of joy or sadness or whether a voice is raised in anger or happy excitement etc. Due to the impaired symbolization capacity, the most serious existential consequences of aphasia appear to be loneliness, feelings of humiliation, inferiority and alienation when efforts to exchange thoughts, feelings, attitudes and experiences with others turn out to be unsuccessful. The interviewees in this study suffered, or had suffered, from different types of aphasia of varying severity. For some, this condition more or less affected all domains of their ability to use and interpret symbols.

The emotional consequences of the loss of one's world of symbols seemed to increase the existential consequences. This was most obvious in one interviewee who lost her son two weeks after suffering a stroke and was unable to mourn for him until she regained her power of speech. She could not cry when she had no words, as if tears are also a part of our commonly shared system of symbols. She and several other interviewees described their difficulties in relating to others, not because they could not speak, but due to feelings of alienation. One of them even felt that the people she encountered were wearing masks. There was only one feeling which all interviewees experienced at an early stage, namely anger.

Over time with increased, but still inadequate, verbal communication, the initial sense of calm disappeared and feelings of self-contempt, suspicion and insecurity emerged. This stage of aphasia was like being in prison. The dreamlike state, the silent "intentional world" described above, was now past over and the interviewees were fully aware of the consequences of losing access to those symbols that constitute connecting links in society. They began to struggle to regain speech and other skills that are connected with symbolization, because they now realised that this was the only way to reclaim their position in society. Their fight was associated with many threats to their self-esteem, but those who were successful were no longer locked inside their bodies. Even if some communication impairments remained at the time ofthe data collection, the interviewees with mainly expressive aphasia could leave their prison having gained an understanding of the importance of communication and interpersonal relations. The most significant sign of successful rehabilitation appears to be the capacity to be completely involved in something other than one's own problems, such as work, caring for one's family, commitment to others with aphasia or political involvement in prioritising rehabilitation for patients with aphasia and so on.

To sum up; the existential meaning of reversible aphasia is that communion, interaction, and interpersonal relations become more important than ever before. Strong elements of continuing aphasia are characterized by a life-and-death struggle to use and/or understand words. Individuals thus affected, even several years after their brain lesion, still find themselves excluded when they fail to express their thoughts and/or guess the meaning of a conversation. In their struggle for existence they need much more time than they are given to talk and/or to fit the puzzle of their fragmented impressions together. During such circumstances it is impossible to direct interest beyond oneself in order to be involved in something other than a struggle for language. The existential meaning of continuing severe aphasia is thus characterized by alienation and loneliness, leaving the individual to find a balance between a fight filled with agony and giving up in order to avoid further humiliation.

The Second Analysis

Professional Aphasia Care

It seems fair to assume that the most devastating consequences of aphasia could be successfully reduced if the principles for care are based not only upon carers' professional opinions, but also on aphasic persons' experiences of good professional care. The following second interpretative analysis is therefore based on data from the same nine informants as were used in the previous part, with focus now on their statements concerning aphasia care. They talked about care that was provided by aphasia therapists, physicians, registered nurses, nursing aides and physiotherapists. In the findings below all professionals are designated "carers". Seven interpretations that illuminated different aspects of aphasia care are presented, followed by a comprehensive understanding. The quotations are excerpted from the data.

Preventing Isolation

This interpretation describes trust in the patient's competence to participate in caring, because a patient with aphasia can be isolated in different ways. The serious effects of impressive aphasia can make communication extremely difficult, although complementing spoken language with gestures and written notes facilitates understanding, and invites the patients to enter a caring relation.

> It is important that the carer writes some words and points to things while talking. That makes it easier for me to guess the meaning of what she is saying.

> With expressive aphasia it is important to continue to talk, even if the patient is unable to reply.

> Talk to us! We do understand!

To prevent isolation it is vital to discover how the patient can best take part in interpersonal interplay. Communication can be facilitated by eliminating disturbances such as noise and reducing the number of persons participating in a conversation. It is most essential to allow the patient sufficient time to concentrate on finding the right words or guessing the meaning of a verbal message. One interviewee with mainly expressive aphasia said:

> When I can't find the right word, the other person can become confused. But given time to close my eyes and search for the right word in my head I can do it.

Another interviewee with mainly impressive aphasia commented:

> It is very hard for me to understand when carers are talking. When I finally find out the meaning of a conversation it has already passed. When people are talking at a normal speed I simply have no chance of following the conversation.

The professional carer's adaptability to the patient's competence and contribution to communication, even if it is non-verbal or very hard to understand, must accord with a unique brain lesion, a unique type of aphasia and, most importantly, a unique person. Carers thus need knowledge and proficiency concerning different types of aphasia in order to understand how to make individual adaptations and help the patient to practice language and break down his/her isolation.

Straightforwardness

This interpretation describes trust in the patient's competence to cope with a situation. The interviewees described how they felt when they were ignored because of their impaired use of language.

> She [the nurse's aid] put the newspaper on my bed, but didn't say anything. After my aphasia she never talked to me again, and avoided eye contact. I understood that she was afraid. Therefore I also became scared.

Such feelings increase when patients are treated as if they cannot cope with their situation. Implicit assumptions about inability can alienate the patient from the caring situation. The opposite is also the case. Being met with straightforwardness makes it easier to cope with a sense of being trapped inside one's body. Straightforwardness also implies an invitation to enter into a communion where the patient recognises that the carer can – and really wants to – meet with him/her as an individual.

> Professional carers ask me if they should supply the right word when an aphasic patient can't find it. I reply that it depends, because we are not all the same. You simply must ask!

This aspect of caring is especially obvious when a carer appears to be uncomfortable with the caring situation or makes light of the problem by saying, for example "you will soon recover", without knowing anything about the severity of the brain lesion.

> Today the physiotherapist said that I talked better than on the
> previous occasion. But on that occasionshe said that I talked well.

If any kind of dishonesty is obvious it is natural to become suspicious. An honest invitation to communicate includes opening up in a direct, straightforward and benevolent manner in an effort to understand the patient. Lack of straightforwardness can be a threat to the patient's self-esteem, and if any kind of dishonesty is recognized it is easy to become suspicious. The reverse is also true. A straightforward approach can reduce anxiety about failing to talk or understand.

Provision for Security

This interpretation describes trust in the patient's competence to feel safe with a carer who really wants to understand, because patients with aphasia can be terrified, even horror-stricken, when they become aware of the consequences of their brain lesion. A secure caring base can alleviate such suffering.

A feeling of security makes it easier for the patient to recognise whether the care is based on genuine interest or a wait-and-see policy. When a patient realises that the carer really wants to know and understand, he/she finds it easier to feel safe. Genuine interest implies that the carer is trying to obtain an overall picture of the patient's communication impairment in order to adapt to it. It does not, however, mean that all patients are emotionally ready to face a sudden, unexpected language defect.

> It was a shock! The physician pointed at the wall and asked me what
> it was. The word wasn't there, I couldn't say anything. Nothing was
> there!

Thus, adaptability that takes each individual patient's reactions into consideration is of vital importance for a secure caring base. It is important to understand when a patient lacks emotional insight into his/her language impairment.

Patients who are not ready to be confronted with their communication impairment can become afraid if the timing of such confrontation is wrong. This kind of awareness on the part of a carer is illuminated by the following statement:

When I arrived in the hospital a nurse talked to me in a warm and calm way. I felt small and helpless. I appreciated her not giving me any information at that moment. She just talked to me in a motherly way.

Recognition of Caring Needs

This interpretation describes trust in the patient's competence to communicate caring needs, because patients with aphasia are vulnerable, as their ability to initiate a dialogue is extremely limited. Professional aphasia care thus includes sufficient time to identify caring needs that are not expressed verbally. It is most important never to allow the patient to feel excluded, isolated and alienated from the caring situation.

> To just sit there mute and stupid, with one's head full of more or less brilliant comments, not being able to make use of them is trying; infernally trying and I became very angry.

If caring includes supporting communication when a patient fails to find the right words or cannot answer at all, the risk of exclusion is reduced. It can also be beneficial to slow down the conversation, complement it with gestures, and help the patient to concentrate by reducing disturbances such as noise.

Yet, the interviewees in the study recalled carers who conversed with each other over their heads. Such attitudes made them feel excluded and humiliated. One interviewee, with expressive aphasia, emphasised:

> We can understand what carers are saying and doing although we cannot always give an answer.

Encouraging Efforts to Practice Language

This interpretation describes trust in the patient's competence to regain lost capacities.The interviewees were angry when they recalled carers who did not support their efforts to communicate. Some carers only recommended rest and taking it easy, leaving them to practise words on their own. A librarian, not a carer, understood one interviewee's silent prayer for something to read, and the textbook she provided helped him to recall words. In another case a patient's twelve-year-old grandson made flash cards with letters and words to be used for communicating caring needs. Aphasia care thus includes language practice during caring activities, as indicated by the following:

One nurse continued to talk to me while she helped me to eat and get dressed. She talked as if she knew that I understood, even though I couldn't answer. That made me feel calm and secure and I knew that she would take good care of me.

A carer who encourages efforts to practise language can increase the patient's motivation to communicate, as well as create trust in the carer's ability to understand caring needs. An invitation to practise language indicates that the carer knows that the patient can understand. Several interviewees were critical of carers who did not take on this responsibility. A further aspect of this failure to take responsibility was that professional carers did not inform the authorities about the need for support from the community services.

Equality

This interpretation describes trust in the patient's competence regarding personal interaction. When patients are confronted with their impairment during conversations with carers they can find themselves in a weak position. Inferiority and lost self-esteem remain for the duration of the aphasia.

The worst was not the handicap itself, but my feelingof being disadvantaged.

When carers do not speak to their patients, or converse with each other over the patients' heads, they relinquish the opportunityto create a working alliance to achieve a shared goal, i.e. communication.

It wasn't nice at all when the nursingaid only told me what to do, but otherwise did not speak to me.

No effort should be spared to create an equal working alliance with the patient. In an autobiography, one interviewee contributed the following example highlighting the importance of equality between carer and patient.

If one talks to a patient on the basis of personal experience one may expose one's own weakness. By so doing the carer raises the patient to her own level. She dares to make the patient equal and at the same time relinquishes some of her power. If she divides her strength the patient's strength increases, because he is no longer the only one who is unsuccessful (Tropp-Erblad 2002 p 35).

Supporting the Maintenance of Identity

This interpretation describes trust in the patient's ability to recognize his or her previous competence, as aphasia can include doubts about who you really are. Such doubts not emanate only from the risk of appearing stupid in the eyes of others, but from a deep anxiety about one's cognitive ability.

> When the aphasia therapist showed me pictures of the brain I became aware of the fact that I didn't understand as well as before. She also asked me to put a pen in a box but I didn't understand her instruction. Now I really had a reason to be scared.

Expressive aphasia is characterised by failure to make other people aware of one's capacity to think and understand. It is therefore a relief when a carer makes it clear that he or she knows that the patient can think. It is also easier to maintain a sense of being the same person as before when the carer refers to the patient's previous competence.

> I couldn't answer, but I think he should have recognised that I understood such matters.

The significance of being aware of the patient's previous competence is also obvious in the following statement. This interviewee is a former physician with severe impressive aphasia. The neurologist told him what had happened by referring to his medical knowledge.

> Then I understood that a part of my brain at the back of my head was more or less gone. It can no longer communicate. Perhaps it is possible for that part of the brain to connect to the undamaged areas. Perhaps an undamaged part that is not yet functional can be activated.

This interviewee had extreme difficulty understanding verbal messages, but was nevertheless able to reflect on his chances of rehabilitation by discussing the situation like a physician. The colleague who helped him to understand referred to his professional identity, which helped him to maintain that part of himself.

Adequate Aphasia Care - Comprehensive Understanding

Patients with aphasia know the meaning of language more fundamentally than they ever did before. They know that with aphasia follows existential shortcomings characterized by the loss of almost everything vivid and important connected with interpersonal relations, leaving them with lost self-esteem, a weak identity and loneliness. A professional carer must thus know how to handle implicit non-verbal questions about who the patient is, as well as feelings of inferiority, frustration and anger.

Trusting the patient's competence while encountering such existential short comings requires a straightforward equal caring relation, which can alleviate inferiority, loneliness and doubts about oneself.

Such encounters are also characterized by the carer's awareness of the patient's possibilities and wishes for support in their efforts to understand and/or to be understood. Adequate professional aphasia care can create a sense of security and community, maintained identity and integrity when the patient is allowed to guide the carers' efforts to discover the best way to practise language.

The most important issue in professional aphasia care is thus to trust the patient's competence while facing existential issues. Such skills can form a secure base that enhances the patient's self-esteem and helps him or her to gain a positive but realistic view of the situation.

The Third Analytic Step

Being Closely Related to a Persons with Aphasia
The third interpretative analysis which follows, is directed towards those closely related to persons with aphasia.

It is based on interviews with seventeen persons with personal experiences of being a spouse, parent or adult son or daughter of a person with severe communication impairments.

The interviewees were encouraged to describe their experiences and their own life situation. Four interpretations emerged, which resulted in a comprehensive understanding that highlights the meaning of being a bridge between a lonely soul and the surrounding world.

Losing Freedom
For close relatives, especially the spouses, communion and cooperation in one's daily life disappear when life abruptly changes after the onset of aphasia. One woman whose husband suffers from severe impressive aphasia says:

I always have to consider the fact that his aphasia makes it frightfully hard for me to be in contact with him, and that leads to loneliness for both of us.

This woman claims to be disabled herself due to her husband's communication impairment. Moreover, he takes her care for granted and is unable to understand that this imprisons them both. Another aphasic man discussed community services without consulting his wife because he wanted her to "take care of everything". Both these women had to take early retirement in order to look after their husbands. Other spouses describe similar dilemmas:

I have to give up what I want to do for myself, because it is a part of the aphasia that they do not want to do anything by themselves, they want company all the time.

He knows what he wants and what he does not want, but I don't exist as a person anymore. He does not understand if I am tired or in pain. No, no, he says if I try to explain. So I am not allowed to have feelings.

I can't give her any responsibility or trust her to do certain things. The whole responsibility lies on my shoulders, in all matters. I often think about the lonely responsibility that makes my life so constrained.

Living with an aphasic person thus means being taken for granted as an informal caregiver, whether or not you have agreed to it. Moreover, none of the interviewees were ever asked by an employee from the community services if they could handle such a situation.

The worst thing that could ever happen to me is to be caught in the situation of being a next-of-kin caregiver after retirement. Worst of all is the humiliation! No one ever asked if they had the right to destroy my life, and that is a deceit on the part of the municipality."

It is devastating always to be restricted by another person's presence, even if it is your husband. You can indeed love a person, but not in a self-sacrificing way. You must have the right to live your own life! This right must be understood by those who decide about community services.

An adult son of a mother with aphasia emphasized the importance of knowledge. He believes that the lack of interest from the community services and political board is due both to a lack of knowledge and to the low status of all illnesses that mostly affect older people. According to him, one manifestation of such an attitude is that aphasia associations rarely receive financial support from the municipality, even when they ask for small contributions. They do not even respond to easy solutions to problems:

> Where I live, in my municipality, many computers are written off every week. It would be easy to load them with programs designed for aphasic people and out them in a meeting place for persons with aphasia. But when I suggested that, they were not interested at all.

Thus, the freedom of close relatives to make choices appears to be lost, especially for those living with the aphasic person. Their lost freedom can be interpreted from two different points of view. The first is the aphasic persons' reduced capacity to understand other people. The second, which greatly contributes to having fewer choices, depends on shortages in the community services. This forces relatives to take on the role of informal caregivers, whether or not they have agreed to it. When the French philosopher Paul Ricoeur (1966) considers the voluntary and the involuntary, he emphasizes that only nature is involuntary. It is indeed impossible to escape the consequences of a brain injury. In this study, the close relatives appear to be well aware of the involuntary nature of aphasia, and they accept it. Yet, it is also obvious that the other aspect of constrained options is voluntary limitations as they are caused by people; here shortfalls in community services.

Choices presuppose the possibility of expressing one's wishes, and a sense of freedom depends on one's possibility to say no. If informal caregivers have that possibility, it seems fair to assume that it would increase their capacity to deal with the difficult and challenging life-situation of being closely related to a person with communication impairments.

Staying

The close relatives in the present study, however, did make one important choice: they stayed. They knew that in similar situations, some people, especially spouses, would not. Some of the interviewees had considered divorce or, in some cases, their workmates had suggested it. Nevertheless, they did not find it a solution as it was impossible for them to leave a loved one, even though a future life together seemed to be filled with problems. The choice to stay is even more obvious to those who are a parent or the adult child of an aphasic person. Yet, irrespective of relationship, they all emphasize that aphasia is the worst possible consequence of a brain injury.

> Aphasia is the most devilish of all the impairments due to stroke. I can accept that she is bound to a wheelchair, but the loss of the ability to speak is unbearable. I don't even know how she feels about it herself. Some linguistic capacity often returns after a while, but then changes in character and temper may occur. Bad temper is often directed towards those who are closest. One husband puts it this way:
> I seem to fuel her anger merely by opening my mouth. She wants to decide everything. She has changed. She came back from her aphasia, but at the same time she did not. Our relationship has become tenser. I think that we would have become closer if she never had that stroke.

One daughter described her mother as formerly a cheerful person, but after a stroke resulting in aphasia, the mother uses bad language.

> My mother always liked to joke. Now she is rough; her words are vulgar and she uses bad language. The first word she said after her stroke was a curse word. I feel bad when I hear her talk like that, and I feel sorry for her because I don't think she means it.

A wife described her despair as her husband is angry with her most of the time:

> It would never have happened before, that he was angry and irritated with me. Initially I told him how sad I was when he was angry with me, but now I have learned to stay calm.

In order to understand the complexity of a person's choice to stay, it is important to consider the fact that apart from all the frustration, sadness and the heavy burden of responsibility, close relatives know that the aphasic person is helpless without them. Therefore, they try to keep in mind that an aphasic person's loss of empathy with other people's needs, as well as their bad temper, is caused by the brain injury. Consequently, it seems reasonable to understand their choice to stay as a duty. Irrespective of whether the decision to stay concerns spouses or parents or adult children, their motto seems to be, "for better or worse".

The French philosopher Emmanuel Levinas (1972) recognizes the acceptance of other people's right to be different from ourselves as an ethical issue. Such an attitude creates a distance from oneself and one's own problems and opens up a space for demands from the other. The duty to stay has an ethical component, as fundamental ethics mostly concern interpersonal relations in general and people close to us in particular. Such ethical assumptions make it possible to put the focus on aphasic person's difficult situation rather than one's own problems. Yet, the close relatives in this study did not talk about duty. They talked about love. Their love conquered all temptations to focus on their own life situation. Love made them reject the idea of another life without the heavy burden of being closely related to a person with communication impairments.

> My colleagues did advise me to divorce her. Nevertheless, I thought that this was something that had hit both of us, and I still love her."

Creating a New Relationship

The person who once existed is partly lost because of the brain injury, and this loss is certainly recognised by the close relatives. Their sorrow does not merely concern the loss of verbal language but of the whole person.

> My dad was always cheerful and chatty. To lose that contact was hard for me.

> I try to get in contact with my father, but it always makes me sad because there is only a part of him left.

> The contact between my mother and me really changed after her aphasia.

> I cried in despair every day the first year. It was a total catastrophe.

Other interpersonal relations, such as those with friends and workmates, dramatically worsen for the affected person. One important part of the close relatives' sad feelings is watching a beloved person's loneliness.

> My wife had many friends before she was ill. Now I believe that they were not real friends, because they never visit her. Nevertheless, I think that she thought that she had a rich social life before her brain injury. Now she doesn't seem to care, but I believe that it remains a disillusionment for her.

The initial period of shock and sorrow gradually changes into an insight into the consequences of aphasia. Gradually the sorrow is worked through, and a new form of relationship emerges. Now it is also possible to see small gleams of light.

> When you can reach into his consciousness, it is possible to recognize that he is still a man of intelligence.

With the use of words so limited, the close relatives work hard to find new ways to communicate. Their inventiveness is huge; questions and guesses are supplemented with gestures, pictures, special noises etc. Sometimes it is easier to sing than talk. However, all such techniques take a lot of time.

> You have to do twice as much in half the time. And you have to be well structured and predictable all the time.

An adult child can be transformed into a parent of his or her own parent after the onset of aphasia. The easiest way out of such a situation can be to concentrate on the practical things that need to be done.

Searching for a new foundation to the relationship can also include new things, such as buying a puppy or listening to music and singing together.

Spouses of aphasic persons spoke of diminished sexual desire, but this did not necessarily mean that their closeness was lost. The longer time spent on understanding each other could in fact lead to a new form of closeness.

> We can sit and hold hands for quite a long time. We cry together and he dries his tears with my hand. So our relationship has changed, but not for the worse.

Some alterations in personality can even lead to changes for the better.

> My husband cares much more about me than before the aphasia. He was very outgoing before he became ill, and he always wanted to do things with his friends. Now he is keener on me."

The initial period of chaos and shock is eventually replaced by one of mourning, followed by a period where it is possible to work through the loss of an earlier relationship and adapt to a new one. Various ways to communicate are tried out and concrete solutions to problems emerge.

The loss turns into a commitment to the person who actually exists, with his or her communication impairments and changes in character. From this follows a new sort of relationship and sometimes a new form of closeness. The creative work of building a new relationship varies, and it fluctuates between despair, exhaustion and acceptance.

Yet, there is something that does not vary. The close relatives search for some remaining essence of the aphasic person's personality. According to the German philosopher Edmund Hussserl's phenomenological philosophy, an essence is described as a structure that makes a phenomenon into that specific phenomenon. This essence illuminates those essential characteristics without which it would not be that particular phenomenon (Dahlberg et.al, 2008), in this case the spouse, parent or adult child who is affected by aphasia. In the close relatives' efforts to find a beloved person's essence, they separate the impairments caused by the brain injury from the characteristics they recognize and recall from the time before the injury. Thus, they search for a genuine personality that still exists. If this essence disappears, the beloved person is gone, but this is not true of any of the cases of this study.

> Yes, he is emotionally shallow now, but his genuine feelings for me and the children are still there.

> I think that her original personality, with a fighting spirit, was a lot of help to her when she started doing things again after her stroke.

> The lovely girl whom I always had is still there. She hugs me when she visits us and when she returns to her nursing home.

> I am pleased to notice that his strong will is intact, because that makes his life endurable.

The close relatives hold on to this essence when reaching the aphasic person even though verbal communication appears impossible. Hence, their new relationship is built on perceptions of the essence of the person who was there before the aphasia.

Growing Strong Together with Others

As previously mentioned, two wives in the study were forced to quit their jobs, and many close relatives had no time for hobbies. Some of them conceal their problems by erecting a façade in order to avoid putting more strain on the family, as they reject the idea that hardships bring a family closer together. Moreover, they have found that the well-developed welfare system and community services in Sweden are a myth.

When discharged from hospital, the close relatives wrongly took it for granted that community services included access to a speech therapist. They were not informed about the limitations in community services, especially after the retirement age in Sweden, i.e. 65 years. The only exception is a spouse who was lucky enough to be included in a research project.

> My husband participated in research and that included a speech therapist three times a week. The speech therapist also talked to me, and it was fantastic to be supported in my communication with him.

Yet, most close relatives in this study were left alone with their fumbling efforts to find new ways to communicate. No professional caregiver ever taught them how to do this. Moreover, socializing with friends or alone also became something of a luxury.

> I feel so good when I have the opportunity to exercise and have coffee and a chat with friends. We discuss books, the theatre, lectures, travels. We all laugh and talk a lot.

> My dream is to be alone in my own home without the obligations to wait on someone all the time. Or, imagine getting a whole night's sleep!

Under such circumstances, being included in new forms of fellowship with other people in the same situation can compensate for the loss of earlier networks and shortcomings in the community services. Membership of aphasia associations thus turns out to be important and valuable.

> In the aphasia association, I meet people who generously share their experiences; this makes me feel very good. It is easier with people in the same situation.

In the aphasia associations, it is easier to take part in activities together with the aphasic persons.

> We enjoy travelling with the aphasia association. Such possibilities are worth a lot. Stimulation is really important, and being able to visit other countries gives a lot. Much of that pleasure remains when we return home. We look at photos together and remember many good things.

It is a relief to find people in the same situations who are able to share their experiences. Such fellowships make it possible to create meaningful activities together with the aphasic person and enjoy moments of relaxation with other close relatives. One important aspect of such encounters is the ability to confirm and receive confirmation in terms of vulnerability as well as an unexpected capacity to deal with problems. Moments to oneself, or with others who are able to understand, make it easier to discover one's own hidden resources.

The British psychoanalyst Donald Winnicot (1971) introduced the idea that moments of active relaxation alone or with others constitute a "potential space" which makes it possible to work through thoughts and feelings. He claims a potential space is an area between the internal life (fantasy) and the external world (reality). In the potential space, we have access to both. This makes it possible to reflect on problems and solve them, initially by imagining possible solutions and then by trying to solve the problem in one's mind. Therefore, having a potential space is an important resource for regaining strength. Fellowship with others in the same situation and the chance to be alone some time appear to increase the possibility of growing stronger than could ever be imagined.

> I have got a new insight. I think that everyone has much greater resources than they know. Human beings seem to have a kind of preparedness for dealing with difficulties but you are not aware of that until something happens.

Being Closely Related to a Person with Aphasia - Comprehensive Understanding

The four interpretations above illuminate how aphasia affects the daily life of close relatives. Their life fluctuates between feeling imprisoned, when they understand that they cannot count on the community services, and growing more confident of their ability to handle the situation. The way to better self-confidence is paved with setbacks, feelings of powerlessness and despair, but also glimpses of hope.

The first analysis in this study shows how people with aphasia feel empty in their internal worlds with no access to adequate words for their own brainwork. Aspects of the same phenomenon appear to be reflected in the close relatives in this third analysis as they become tied to an aphasic person and lose the opportunities to do things with other people or by themselves. Leaving the aphasic person alone is not an option, because that would mean leaving him or her empty both in internal and external sense. Therefore, they strive to find new things or new ways of doing old things together. During that process, they create a new form of relationship.

Being closely related to an aphasic person thus seems to comprise existential issues, which in turn raise identity questions such as: Who was I before? Who am I now, when my chances to choose my own way of life are gone? What will I be in the future? Will I always be reduced to an informal caregiver?

One tentative explanation for such an identity crisis is that close relatives seem to take on the part of acting as an extension of the aphasic person's body and mind. According to Maurice Merleau-Ponty (1989), our "lived bodies" can be extended by using *things* that increase our possibilities to participate in the surrounding world. Some well-known examples from that element of Merleau-Ponty's philosophy are a cane or a pen that are experienced as the prolongation of an arm or hand, or music instruments or cars as extensions of one's body.

Merleau-Ponty also stresses that all forms of illness result in changed access to the world because of one's lost abilities and interruptions to harmonic living. This is certainly true when the most important part of the body, i.e. the brain, is struck by illness. Aphasic people find themselves in a situation where it is necessary to rely on others as extensions of their body and mind. Being closely related to an aphasic person consequently includes a tendency to be used as a *thing*, in the sense that Merleau-Ponty suggests or, to put it more concretely, as a bridge between a lonely soul and the surrounding world.

A common denominator in the four themes described above thus concerns new ways of viewing oneself. The close relatives gain an acceptance of their current life-situation, that is beyond their earlier capacity. They decide to stay and continue to serve and love. In doing so, they also make a knowing which gives them confidence in their self-image as a person who does not desert a loved one.

The Synthesizing Analysis

Aphasia Care and Support- a Mutual Concern and a Shared Responsibility

The first part of this study illuminated how a person with aphasia copes with existential loneliness and feelings of alienation in social settings. The possibilities to be part of the communion appear not only to differ according to the type, severity and reversibility of the aphasia itself but also to other persons' wishes and capacity to interact in spite of obvious obstacles to communication. The second part described how professional carers can be of assistance in the struggle to regain communication skills by trusting the patients' competence. The third part was directed to something often neglected, the close relatives who are informal caregivers. The meaning of that was interpreted as being a bridge between a lonely soul and the surrounding world.

Putting one's feelings into words is a well-known psychotherapeutic basis for achieving awareness of one's motives and choices (cf. Blanck and Blanck, 1974). According to Gadamer (1996), words are "foodfor thought", and humanity would have been unable to construct cultural traditions without the miracle of language. A further important aspect of language was introduced during the 1930s by George Herbert Mead (1934). According to him, human communication is a consequence of role-taking. In order to communicate, every person must be able to assume the role of the other and address him or her in a language that both understand. In other words, we cannot begin to communicate without making assumptions about the internal operation of the mind of the other. Role-taking thus carries with it enormous social and personal benefits. It allows genuine interaction, and permits cooperation and compromise as well as making possible a depth of interpersonal relations that would otherwise be unattainable. This is also important for our capacity to use and understand symbols and signs in accordance with our cultural tradition.

Thus, aphasic people are certainly vulnerable, as their ability to enter into a dialogue on their own initiative can be extremely limited. Therefore, conversation in line with their communication impairment, is essential for their ability to participate in social life. In this process it is important not to conceive of language as a form of adherence to fixed rules. The real miracle of language is to be found when the aphasic person discovers the meaning in the words of someone else and is able to express meaning themselves.

Many health care theorists also emphasize the power of interaction between a professional caregiver and patient. According to Peplau (1991), a professional carer must also understand his or her own behaviour in order to help patients to understand how their individual disabilities and impairments affect their situation.

Apart from a few studies within healthcare science, reflections on interpersonal relations in the care of patients with aphasia appear to be quite rare. Coping with the most devastating consequences of aphasia seems nevertheless to be related to interpersonal relations. It thus seems reasonable to suppose that inferiority, self-contempt and suspicion can be successfully reduced by means of positive communication, interaction and a sense of community. Thus, a caregiver's capacity to assist in finding that symbols function for communication is of vital importance for patients with continuing aphasia.

Some of the professional carers referred to by the informants in the second part of this study appear to have been able to create a starting point for acceptance and working through the dreadful experience of losing the world of symbols, by trusting and assisting the patient's competence to deal with such losses. One question, however, remains. How can another person know about individual existential issues if the aphasic person cannot put them into words? There seems to be an urgency in pondering whether language has an existential meaning in itself, or if the meaning of language is best understood by those who have experienced losing it?

According to Martin Heidegger's existential philosophy the breakdown of a tool momentarily highlights it's presence (i.e. *Being* in Heidegger's terminology) in the "world" in which it exists (Heidegger 1998). If this is the case even with such a fundamental "tool" as language its full meaning is visible to those affected by aphasia, while it is hidden from everyone who has not had such an experience.

This is, however, a poor consolation to those affected. Frustration, anxiety and anger seem to be important aspects of the struggle to regain the capacity to communicate, as they contribute to the disappearance of the illusory initial calmness, thus making room for a fighting spirit. Even those with continuing aphasia appear to be helped by their frustration, as it serves as a driving force that motivates them to practise speech and written language.

But for those closely related, especially spouses, easily awakened frustration and anger can be experienced as frightening personality changes. When the brain injury also includes impairment of the skill to understand and show an interest in other people the strain on close relatives is further increased.

In the first analyse this was exemplified by the aphasic persons' experience of being empty inside their head. Difficulties in improvising thoughts and indulgence in daydreams made them lonely, not only in social settings but also in an internal sense. That, in turn, could increase their need for another person's constant presence.

The same issue was illuminated from another aspect when close relatives were interviewed. Spouses in particular claimed to be trapped without the chance to do anything for and by themselves. They had turned into extensions of the afflicted person's body and mind.

Yet, such consequences of the brain damage were not the most frustrating part of the close relatives' lost freedom, which was the lack of support from community services. Hence, there are consequences to being closely related to an aphasic person that appear to be unnecessary; they depend on an insufficient community service. If close relatives' fundamental rights to decide how to manage their own lives are attended to, it will probably enhance their ability to assist a family member with communication impairments. It is therefore important in providing professional help to include issues concerning how to balance their responsibility against the responsibility of professional carers and community service.

It is thus reasonable to conclude that aphasia management practice, in the long run has to be a shared responsibility. Principles for this can be outlined under the following headings:

- The first task is to provide the aphasic person with a secure base,consisting of *both* professional support and informal caregiving of close relatives. The secure base can form the starting point for exploring possibilities for interpersonal communication with help from a trusted companion who continues to talk even when answers are lacking.
- The second task is to encourage the aphasic person to consider how current perceptions and expectations can make room for a fighting spirit. Some require time, while others immediately start searching for a way out of their verbal prison. For the first group the spirit can be even more paralysed than the body, but for all it is extremely urgent to prevent further isolation that will make them withdraw even more.
- The third task is to assist the aphasic person by encouraging their efforts to talk about things that really matter. If encouraged to express personal reactions and feelings, such as frustration and anger, they may find it easier to maintain integrity and identity. Others must not take rejections personally. When an aphasic person is angry the professional caregiver or the close relative has an opportunity to practice stepping back and analysing the situation.
- The fourth task concerns the importance of facilitating communication by helping nature and simply continuing to talk. During small talk it is important that the aphasic person is given enough time and that other disturbing factors are minimized. It can

also be productive to complement words with gestures or written words if it helps to make understanding easier.

- The fifth task is to spare no efforts to understand the aphasic person's existential situation. This requires a reflective stance that makes it possible to find new creative methods to communicate that accord with the different types of aphasia. This is extremely important because regaining the ability to communicate can reduce humiliation and feelings of alienation and loneliness.

- The sixth task is to enable aphasic persons to recognize that theirself-images derive from the painful experience of losing the world of symbols. Inside they are the same as before, and it is important that others show that they recognize this. It is thus important for professional carers and close relatives, as well as personnel from community services, to reflect upon how to help the aphasic person to maintain a clearly defined self, by referring to their previous competence.

- The synthesising step in this study makes it reasonable to suggest that community service should include education in speech training and counselling on how to handle booth practical and existential matters. Target groups for such measures are not only aphasic persons and their close relatives but also the personnel employed by community services to support those families.

References

Andersson, S. and Fridlund, B. (2002). The Aphasic Person's Views of the Encounter with Other People: A Grounded Theory Analysis.*Journal of Psychiatric and Mental Health Nursing, 9,* 285-292.

Berthier, ML. (2005). Poststroke Aphasia: Epidemilogy, Pathophysiology, and Treatment. *Drugs and Aging, 22,* 2, 163-82.

Blake, H., Lincoln, N.B., and Clark, D.D. (2003). Caregiver strain in spouses of stroke patients. Clinical Rehabilitation, 17, 312-317.

Blanck, G., and Blanck, R. (1974). *Ego psychology – Theory and Practice*New York: Columbia University Press.

Bäckström, B., and Sundin, K. (2007). The Meaning of Being a Middle-aged Close Relative of a Person Who Has Suffered Stroke, One Month after Discharge from a Rehabilitation Clinic. *Nursing Inquiry, 14,* 243-254.

Charon, JM. (1989). *Symbolic Interactionism. An Introduction, an Interpretation, an Integration.* Prentice Hall, Englewood Cliffs.

Cunningham, R. (1998). Counselling Someone with Severe Aphasia: an Explorative Case Study. *Disability and Rehabilitation, Sep, 20,* 9, 346-54.

Dahlberg, K., Dahlberg, H., and Nyström, M. (2008). *Reflective Lifeworld Research.* Lund: Studentlitteratur.

Dahlin, A. (1997) *Den onödiga proppen (The unnecessary thrombosis).* Visby: Visby författarförlag.

Freud, A. (1966). The writings of Anna Freud. Vol II *The ego and the mechanism of defence.* New York: International Hallmark Press.

Freud, S. (1968). *Drömtydning (The interpretation of dreams).* Stockholm: Bonniers.

Gadamer, H-G. (1996). *The Enigma of Health.* Stanford California: StanfordUniversity Press.

Gadamer, H-G. (1997). *Truth and Method.* Second Revised Edition. New York: The Continuum Publishing Company.

Heidegger, M. (1998). *Being and Time.* (J. Macquarrie and E. Robinson. Trans.) Oxford Blackwells.

Husserl, E. (1970). *Logical Investigations: Vol.1.* Prolegomena to pure logic. London: Routledge and Kegan Paul.

Lau, A., and Mckenna, K. (2001). Conceptualizing Quality of Life for Elderly People with Stroke. *Disability Rehabilitation, 23,* 227-38.

Levinas, E. (1972). *Humanisme de l'autre homme.*(Humanism and the other man) Paris: Fata Morgana.

Mead, G.H. (1934). *Mind, Self and Society.* Chicago: University of Chicago Press.

Merleau-Ponty, M. (1989). *Phenomenology of Perception.* Translated by Colin Smith. London: Routledge.

Nyström, M. (2006). Aphasia- An Existential Loneliness: A Study on the Loss of the World of Symbols. *International Journal of Qualitative Studies on Health and Wellbeing,* 1, 38-49.

Nyström, M. (2009) Professional Aphasia Care – Trusting the Patient's Competence while Facing Existential Issues. *Journal of Clinical Nursing,18,* 2503-2510.

Nyström, M. (2011). A Bridge Between a Lonely Soul and the Surrounding World: A Study on Existential Consequences of Being Closely Related to a Person with Aphasia. *International Journal of Qualitative Studies on Health and Wellbeing,* 6: 7911-DOI: 10.3402/qhw.v6i4.7911.

O'Connell, B., Baker, L., Prosser, A. (2003). The Educational Needs of Carers of Stroke Survivors in Acute and Community Settings: Are They Being Addressed? *Journal of Neuroscience Nursing, 5*, 21-28.

Peplau, H. (1991). *Interpersonal Relations in Nursing*. London: MacMillan Education Ltd.

Ricoeur, P. (1966). *Freedom and Nature: the Voluntary and the Involuntary*. North Western University Press.

Ricoeur, P. (1976). *Interpretation theory. Discourse and the Surplus of Meaning*. Fort Worth Texas Christian University Press.

Robinson, R.G. (2002). Psychiatric Management of Stroke. *Psychiatric Annals, 32*, 121-127.

Sawatzky, J,E., and Fowler-Kerry, S. (2003). Impact of Care Giving: Listening to the voice of informal caregivers. *Journal of Psychiatry Mental health Nursing, 10*, 277-86.

Sundin, K., and Jansson, L. (2003). 'Understanding and being understood' as a creative caring phenomenon – in care of patients with stroke and aphasia. Journal of Clinical Nursing, 12, 107-116.

Tacke, D. (1999). Nursing Care of Patients with Aphasia – a literature study. *Phlege, 12*, 95-100.

Tooth, L., McKenna,. K., Barnett, A., Prescott, C., and Murphy, S. (2005). Caregiver Burden, Time Spent, Caring and Health Status in the First 12 Months Following Stroke. Brain Injury, 19, (12), 963-974.

Tropp-Erblad, I. (2002). *Katt börjar på S (Cat begins with S)*.Afasiförbundet i Sverige: Författarnas bokmagasin.

Wallengren, C., Friberg, F., and Segesten, K. (2008). Like a Shadow – on Becoming a Stroke Victim's Relative.*Scandinavial Journal of Caring Sciences, 22*, 48-55.

van der Gaag, A., Smith, L., Davis, S., Moss, B., Cornelius, V., Laing, S., Mowles,C. (2005).Therapy and Support Services for People with Long-term Stroke and Aphasia and their Relatives: a Six-month Follow-up Study. *Clinical Rehabilitation,* 19, 4, 372-380

Winnicot, D. (1971). *Playing and Reality*New York: Basic Books.

Maria Nyström is a Registered Nurse, Master in Psychology and Doctor in Nursing Pedagogy. Since 2006 she is Professor in Caring Science at the University of Borås in Sweden. She has a special interest in Qualitative Research Methods, and her Research Focus on Existential Issues related to Sickness and Health.

In: Aphasia   ISBN: 978-1-62257-681-4
Editors: E. Holmgren, E.S. Rudkilde © 2013 Nova Science Publishers, Inc.

Chapter II

Aphasia: Pharmacological and Non-Pharmacological Management

Muhammad Rizwan Sardar,[1]* Muhammad Maaz Iqbal[2]
and Wajeeha Saeed[2]#
[1]Lankenau Medical Center, Main Line Heart Center, Wynnewood, PA, US
[2]Montefiore Medical Center, New York, NY, US

Abstract

From the simplistic explanations of Wernicke's and Broca's, to the latest investigative headways made into the understanding of intricacies involved in the use of the spoken and written words; modern science is still in the process of understanding Aphasias. The use of radiological and pathological diagnostic modalities in the study of language deficits has helped in the recognition of two categories of aphasias. The acute and sub-acute presentations seen mostly in association with cerebrovascular accidents, CNS infections, and head trauma shows involvement of specific parts of the perisylvian language network which is located in the

---

* Lankenau Medical Center, Main Line Heart Center. 100 E Lancaster Avenue, MOB E 558, Wynnewood PA 19096. Ph.: 347-327-2734, Fax: 718-904-4169. E-mail: sardarr@mlhs.org, msardar@montefiore.org.
# Montefiore Medical Center. 1825 Eastchester Road, Rm W 1-95, Bronx, NY 10461. 718-904-3293.

left hemisphere in majority of right as well as left-handed individuals. Based upon the evaluation of spontaneous speech, naming, comprehension, repetition, reading and writing, and diagnostic imaging these aphasias are divided into central aphasias and the disconnection syndromes. The central aphasias, namely Wernicke's and Broca's are due to damage of the two classical, though not anatomically discrete language centers bearing the same names. The disconnection syndromes are a result of damage to areas of the language network other than the classical centers and include Transcortical and Conduction Aphasias among others. The slowly progressive aphasias caused by neurodegenerative diseases are referred to as Primary progressive aphasias (PPA). In order to simplify understanding of these aphasias and thereby help find cures these aphasias have recently been classified into the agrammatic, semantic, and logopenic variants. Management and prognostic issues pertaining exclusively to language disruption are widely studied in the aphasias with actual presentation. The mainstay of treatment is speech and language therapy; however some drugs are also showing promise especially when combined with language therapy. In post-stroke aphasic patients there is a strong correlation between initial severity and eventual recovery. Although most improvement occurs in the first few months, late language therapy has also shown benefit. Ongoing research also points to the potential utility of transcranial magnetic and electric stimulation for the treatment of certain aphasias.

Introduction

Aphasia is an acquired impairment of production or comprehension of language or both resulting from damage to the language network in the brain [1-3].

Beginning in the nineteenth century with the Daxs' almost-forgotten theories and Broca's revolutionizing articles, our understanding of normal language and its impairment has come a long way [4,5]. Although the concept of language centers is still found in clinical literature, it has been widely accepted that these centers are not circumscribed islands but various interconnected parts of the whole language network [6, 7]. In the majority of people, right-handed as well as left-handed (although to a lesser degree) this language network is located in the frontal, temporal and parietal Perisylvian areas of the left cerebral hemisphere [8, 9]. Aphasia secondary to lesions in the right hemisphere in right-handed individuals is rare and referred to as the Crossed aphasia [10].

It is worthy of notice that although impairments in the use of the spoken and written word have been vastly studied, however, the communication using gestures remains relatively less well incorporated into our overall understanding of aphasias [11].

Classification

The radiologic-pathologic correlation of the onset, progression and associated symptomatology of specific deficits in language perception and or production has led to the recognition of two broad but distinct clinical patterns of aphasia.

The acute and sub-acute presentations are seen with directly or indirectly demonstrable involvement of specific parts of the left Perisylvian language network. These aphasias may be "central aphasias", resulting from damage to the two famous language centers, namely Wernicke's and Broca's, or the result of damage to areas of the language network other than the classical centers, the latter being termed the "Disconnection syndromes". [12,13]

On the other hand, chronic aphasias caused by neurodegenerative diseases show only atrophic changes on brain imaging and are dealt with under the umbrella term "Primary Progressive Aphasia" (PPA). The classification of PPA into the Agrammatic, Semantic, and Logopenic variants is a recent and important development to streamline efforts for the formulation of diagnostic criteria and management guidelines for this heterogeneous group of disorders [14].

The Classic Aphasias

These aphasias have been studied for over a century now and became the starting point of the intensive and revealing debate and research in the evolving field of the Aphasiology. They include Broca's, Wernicke's, Global, Conduction, Transcortical, Anomic and Subcortical aphasias.

1. Broca's Aphasia
Originally described by the French physician Pierre Broca in 1861, this is primarily a deficit in speech production with relatively preserved language comprehension [7,15, 16]. Repetition and naming are impaired as well [16]. It must be borne in mind that comprehension is only relatively preserved and this

becomes evident when the patient fails to understand long and complex sentences [7, 17].

The deficit in speech production is manifested by varying combinations of reduced phrase length, agrammatic sentence production, impaired melody of speech and decreased words per minute (10 to 15 words per minute compared to the normal rate of 100 to 115 words per minute) [6,16,18]. Spontaneous speech displays somewhat better utterance of generally familiar words e.g. *hi* and patients feels relatively better at singing a familiar song than at spontaneous speech [12, 18]. These deficits combine giving rise to the so-called telegraphic speech. In most severe forms there may be absolutely no understandable speech production with only one or few repetitive words or utterances accounting for the whole speech output The patient is aware of the deficit, and the inability to convey the desired message via normal speech leads to visible consternation displayed by the patient's facial expressions and body gestures [12].

Despite the above mentioned speech output impairments, these patients generally succeed in conveying some part of the desired message, as the words which they do complete are clearly directed towards the specific idea or thought that is meant to be conveyed.

Neurological Damage and Causes

Broca's aphasia results from lesions involving the posterior part of the left Inferior frontal gyrus; this includes the Broca's area (Brodmann areas 44 and 45) and extends into adjacent parts of the Perisylvian frontal and Insulary cortices [2, 16, 19].

The most frequent cause of this damage is embolic occlusion of the superior division of the left Middle cerebral artery (MCA) with the most typical neurological symptoms being displayed in the acute phase [19-21].

Other causes include hemorrhagic strokes and cerebral space occupying lesions (e.g. tumors and abscesses) affecting the same cortical areas [12].

Associated Features

As expected of impediments involving the superior division of left MCA, most cases are accompanied by right-sided upper limb and right-sided facial weakness Damage which is exclusively limited to the Broca's area or some part of it results in purely motor articulatory impairments which have been referred to as Aphemia [2] or Apraxia of speech [16]. Due to its presentation Broca's aphasia has also been referred to as nonfluent, anterior, motor or expressive aphasia [18,22,23].

2. Wernicke's Aphasia

Originally described by the German physician Carl Wernicke in 1874, Wernicke's Aphasia refers to a primary deficit in both spoken and written language comprehension with paraphasic, neologistical yet fluent speech output [16, 24,25]. Naming and repetition are impaired with repetition being as paraphasic and neologistic as spontaneous speech. Reading and writing skills are impaired as well [12].

These deficits in language comprehension and output are manifested by effortless, normally intoned spontaneous speech which is rendered relatively meaningless by excessive function words (pronouns, articles, prepositions etc.), paraphasias or word substitutions which may be full (semantic paraphasias e.g. fork for knife) or partial (phonemic paraphasias e.g. pymarid for pyramid) and utterance of neologisms or bizarre non-words [2,16,18,23]. These three defects combine giving rise to the so-called jargon speech [26].

These patients are unable to comprehend their own meaningless speech as well as others' speech and are at the same time totally unaware of this inability. In comparison with Broca's aphasia these patients may suffer anxiety but to a much lesser extent. Their frustration seemingly stems from others' inability to understand their speech, the incomprehensibility of which they are unaware of themselves owing to the lack of insight. Wernicke's Aphasia has also been referred to as fluent, posterior, sensory, or receptive aphasia [18, 22, 23].

Neurological Damage and Causes

Wernicke's aphasia results from lesions involving the posterior part of the left Superior temporal gyrus including the classically described Wernicke's area (Brodmann area 22) with damage usually extending into adjacent parts of the Supramarginal and Angular gyri of the left inferior Parietal lobe [26].

The most frequent cause of this damage is infarction of the inferior division of the left Middle cerebral artery (MCA) [16, 19]. Other causes include hemorrhagic strokes, severe head trauma and cerebral space occupying lesions (e.g. tumors and abscesses) affecting the same cortical areas [12, 18]. Wernicke's aphasia has also been reported as an outcome of patients presenting initially with global aphasia [27].

Associated Features

Most cases are accompanied by right homonymous hemianopia or right superior quadrantanopia [12].

3. Global Aphasia

This can be understood as a combination of the upper two aphasias and is characterized by profound involvement of all aspects of language perception and production including comprehension, spontaneous speech, naming, repetition, reading and writing [16].

Neurological Damage and Causes

Global Aphasia results from lesions involving large parts of the left Perisylvian language network including Broca's area, Wernicke's areas and adjacent parts of the inferior parietal lobule [16, 19].

It is usually caused by a large embolic occlusion of the left Less frequent causes include hemorrhagic strokes and cerebral space occupying lesions (e.g. tumors and abscesses) affecting the whole language network [18]. Transient global aphasia is also reported in postictal state, metabolic disturbances like hypoglycemia, hyponatremia and transient reversible stress induced cardiomyopathy. [18,29, 137]

Associated Features

As expected of large occlusions involving the left MCA most cases are accompanied by right hemiplegia, right facial weakness and right homonymous hemianopia [2,12].

Global Aphasia without Hemiparesis (GAWH)

This is an interesting uncommon clinical entity in which the patients show global language impairments without any facial and body weakness. GAWH has been reported with multiple embolic occlusions of various branches of the left MCA as well as with single large occlusions. Less frequent causes include hemorrhagic strokes and cerebral metastases affecting the language network [27].

4. Conduction Aphasia

Both Wernicke and Lichtheim hypothesized that the disruption of neuronal connections between the two language centers (Broca's and Wernicke's) would cause a distinct set of symptoms and Wernicke coined the term "Conduction Aphasia" [24,30,31].

These patients have problems in repetition with meaningful, relatively fluent, slightly paraphasic (phonemic paraphasias [2]) speech with relatively intact comprehension of both spoken and written language [16]. The patient is aware of the problem and makes several attempts at self-correction characteristically, though not universally, producing a pattern termed "conduite d'approche" e.g., *"splant, plant, plants, pants"* for pants [16,32].

Although naming, reading and writing tasks also disclose impairments, the impairment in repetition is markedly disproportionate.

Neurological Damage and Causes

In line with the earlier theories proposing damage to interconnecting pathways, it was believed that this aphasia is caused by damage to a white matter tract running between Wernicke's and Broca's areas called the Arcuate Fasciculus [33]. However the following considerations have led many specialists to search for other regions complicit in the causation of this aphasia:

- Damage to sites other than the Arcuate fasciculus including the left Superior temporal gyrus and the supramarginal gyrus has been demonstrated in conduction aphasic patients with a degree of consistency [34, 35].
- Multiple reports have been made of cases with repetition defects (one of the hallmarks of Conduction Aphasia) but with lesions sparing the Arcuate fasciculus [36, 37].
- Absence of conduction aphasia in patients with damaged or missing arcuate fasciculus [38,39].

5. Transcortical Aphasias

Being any one of the sensory, motor and mixed varieties the Transcortical aphasias are characterized by relatively preserved repetition [2, 16].

Originally described by the German physicians Wernicke and Lichtheim, the Transcortical Aphasias were elaboratedin detail by Goldstein who also referred it to using the phrase "isolation of the speech area" and traced the origin of the term"Transcortical" to Wernicke [40, 41].

A. Transcortical Motor Aphasia

With the exception of intact repetition, the motor variety is similar to Broca's aphasia with nonfluent speech output and relatively intact language comprehension [2, 16].

Neurological Damage and Causes

This is most commonly seen in infarcts of the left anterior cerebral artery (ACA) or the left ACA-MCA watershed area which typically damage the regions surrounding Broca's area thereby sparing or isolating it [16,42,43].

Associated Features

Signs which may give a hint towards the occluded portion in appropriate clinical settings include apathy and right sided hemiparesis [44].

B. Transcortical Sensory Aphasia

With the exception of intact repetition, the sensory variety is similar to Wernicke's aphasia with fluent, paraphasic speech output and impaired comprehension of written and spoken language [2, 16].

Neurological Damage and Causes

This is most commonly seen in infarcts of the left Posterior cerebral artery (PCA) or the left PCA-MCA watershed territory resulting in isolation of Wernicke's area [45].

Associated Features

Right visual field deficits may be seen in these cases [16].

C. Transcortical Mixed Aphasia

With the exception of intact repetition, this is quite similar to global aphasia [16].

Neurological Damage and Causes

This usually results from multiple emboli occluding the anterior (ACA-MCA) and posterior (PCA-MCA) cerebral watershed areas [46]. Other causes include anoxia and carbon monoxide poisoning [12].

Associated Features

As might be expected this aphasia may be accompanied by right Hemiparesis and/or right hemianopia [16, 46].

6. Anomic Aphasia

While naming difficulties of varying severities form part of the symptom-complex in various aphasias, "Anomic aphasia" is designated when naming of objects, persons, events, and things is selectively impaired, with comprehension, spontaneous speech, repetition, reading and writing skills being preserved [16, 47].

Although pure anomic aphasia is a rare entity interesting phrases like "word-finding difficulties" [48] and "tip-of-the-tongue" [49] situations have been used by experts to describe it. Owing to the specific defect in naming, spontaneous speech is fluent but circumlocutory and paraphasic [47].

The patient is aware of the deficit and shows obvious effort to find the correct words [48].

Neurological Damage and Causes

The part of the language network damaged has not been specifically localized. Different reports showing involvement of the left anterior inferior temporal lobe left middle temporal gyrus, and the left temporo-occipital junction have been made [48-51].

Anomic aphasia has mostly been attributed to head trauma, metabolic encephalopathy, strokes and brain surgery while Herpes simplex encephalitis has also been reported as a rare cause [12,48].

7. Subcortical Aphasias

Aphasias have traditionally been considered a cortical problem [52]. Therefore the reporting of heterogeneous aphasias, defying the specific patterns described above, in patients suffering from subcortical lesions started an exciting new phase in this remarkable field of aphasiology [53-55].

While the specific role of subcortical structures in speech generation has been acknowledged, there have been studies which strongly raise the possibility that the cortical deficits in the presumed subcortical aphasic patients simply remained undetected due to the lack of modalities like SPECT, PET and advanced MRI at the time of reporting [52,56-58].

Treatment and Prognosis of Classic Aphasias

While it can be said that much progress has been made in our understanding of aphasias, similar progress may not be claimed in the development of effective treatments for this disorder at this time. Generally speaking any reversible causes of brain damage or dysfunction should be addressed first and foremost e.g. potential reperfusion of hypoxic brain tissue, treatment of any hypoglycemia or electrolyte imbalance, steroids for cerebral edema or possible surgical removal of any intra- or extra-axial mass lesions etc. Over time the development and co-existence of depression is common and should be regularly evaluated [59,60]. Upon detection of depression or any other psychiatric illness expert advice and care might be required.

Since about a quarter to a third of stroke survivors suffer from aphasia it would not be surprising to find that aphasia outcomes and treatment approaches have been most widely studied in post-stroke aphasic patients [61,62]. Various techniques and approaches are being studied and developed by neuroscience researchers, speech pathologists and therapists and neurologists aiming to cure or at least ameliorate this problem to an acceptable functional status. Only language therapy is the validated treatment at present [63]. Pharmacologic interventions are being rapidly tested and transcranial stimulation (magnetic and electric) remains the least investigated potential treatment option for aphasic patients [64].

Intensive Speech and Language Therapy

Although showing variable effectiveness from highly to minimally effective in different reports, Speech and language therapy remains the mainstay of aphasia treatment [63,65]. This therapy has especially been shown to be effective in the acute stage of the aphasia, although benefit has also been reported if it is started in the chronic stage [63, 66]. Moreover it has now been established that short-term intense therapy sessions have superior efficacy when compared to spread-out treatment plans [63, 67].

Customization of Therapy

Vascular aphasias present in various different forms varying in the type of disability as well as the severity. Coupling this with the diverse patient population coming from all the socioeconomic strata of society with their different possible minimal functional target levels creates a wide array of factors which have to be considered while instituting speech therapy. The therapist and neurologist have the tedious task of making treatment regimens that will not only theoretically improve the functional status of the patient but also ensure compliance [68]. It is, therefore, imperative that the therapy be customized to the individual patient's needs, disabilities, motivation level and stamina [69].

Constraint-Induced Aphasia Therapy (CIAT)

As a natural response to this acquired disability aphasic patients adapt to the situation and develop strategies to bypass their deficits and exceedingly try to communicate via use of simplest possible phrases that they can utter or through gestures [70]. Though this is a clear attempt at self-rehabilitation, one harmful consequence of this reaction is the nonuse of all spared language abilities resulting in the actual recovery falling short of its full potential [71].

The aim of CIAT is to help the patient achieve highest levels of potential recovery. As the name indicates CIAT involves intense therapy sessions while minimizing the use of non-verbal communications. This approach seems to be very promising in efficacy as well as cost-effectiveness and needs to be studied at much larger levels [72-74].

Melodic Intonation Therapy

The use of music and singing sessions to improve speech output is being specifically studied in Broca's aphasia patients who demonstrate a lesser loss of singing skills at baseline as compared to spontaneous speech [12].

Pharmacologic Therapy

The manipulation of neurotransmitters in the brain especially in the regions surrounding the lesioned site seems to be a potential area of exploration for possible remedies [75]. However no agent has been unequivocally proven so far to be practically effective and safe in post- stroke aphasic patients [76]. Some drugs which might become useful in the future include:

- Piracetam combined with speech therapy has been shown to improve both speech production and comprehension [77].
- Donepezil is a cholinergic agent which has been shown to give sustained benefit up to six months after discontinuation [78].
- Memantine is an N-methyl-d-aspartate receptor antagonist with a good safety profile and has shown very promising results when combined with the already established CIAT [79].

Prognosis

The deleterious effects of aphasia on the life of the patient are both intensive and extensive. The disruptions caused in the patient's life range from the obvious problems in maintaining interpersonal relationships and meeting professional requirements to overt or covert depression in the patients themselves or in their caregivers [59,80,81].At least some degree of recovery of language function is shown by a large majority of post-stroke aphasic patients [82]. Regardless of the specific type of aphasia left-handed individuals tend to show better recovery patterns than right-handed people [18] and sparing of Wernicke's area is associated with better outcomes [12].

Although occasional recovery has been shown to occur up to several years after the initial insult, significant spontaneous recovery has been shown to occur mainly with in the first three months [78, 83, 84]. This also falls in line with the observation of some experts that maximum treatment benefit is also derived by instituting language therapy early in the course of the impairment [63, 66]. An interesting explanation put forth for this faster early recovery [85] is that the perilesional environment at that time, with its increased growth factor content, presents a promotive milieu for neuronal and synaptic recovery [86,87].

A strong correlation exists between the severity of the initial insult and eventual recovery in most of the cases [88-90].

Primary Progressive Aphasia (PPA)

Primary Progressive Aphasia (PPA) is a clinical syndrome characterized by progressive language impairment with the conspicuous absence of other cognitive impairments like visuospatial or memory skills for the first two years and presence of only atrophic changes on imaging of the left perisylvian language network [14].In essence the generalized foci of affected brain tissue dealt with in the classic aphasias are not applicable to PPA, which results from perpetual neurodegeneration with simultaneous neuronal reorganization in the affected areas [14].

As may also be inferred from the preceding statement PPA is a disease of advanced age [91, 92]. Owing to the continuous increase in life expectancy [93] and its implicit health care cost burden [94], definitive diagnosis and treatment of this entity has become an object of paramount importance for neurological experts as well as health care administrators and policy makers.

PPA has been further categorized into three distinct variants.

1. Agrammatic Variant (PPA-G)

The characteristically encountered problems in this variant include slow spontaneous speech with [14,95-97]:

- Anomia.
- progressive inability to produce properly structured sentences, the sentences being devoid of the small words ("determiners") that precede nouns in normal speech, like *the* professor, *a* school, *a bit of* mustard, *that* lady.
- Improper word-order in sentences.

These combined with the initially less obvious decreasing speech fluency lead to considerable disability over time. However, it is noteworthy that even in the advanced stages of the condition there is relative preservation of comprehension. Patients are aware of their language impairment [98-99].

Imaging Characteristics

Following patterns of atrophic changes have been noted:

- In the left posterior inferior frontal gyrus (Broca's area), Insula, premotor and supplementary motor areas [100].
- A smaller proportion of cases have shown generalized left perisylvian atrophy [101].
- Normal neuroimaging has also been reported [102].

Neuropathology

This is variable, however, histopathology of a number of cases of PPA-G demonstrates patterns consistent with Pick's disease or corticobasal degeneration (CBD) pathology with neurons containing a microtubule-associated protein tau (MAPT) [102,103].

Associated Features

Many cases with agrammatic variant of PPA show extra pyramidal features of corticobasal degeneration (CBD) and progressive supranuclear palsy (PSP) [104, 105] e.g. bradykinesia and gaze palsy during the course of the disease. Limb apraxia has also been reported [106].

PPA-G may also be referred to as nonfluent variant PPA (nfvPPA) [91] or Progressive nonfluent aphasia (PNFA) [107].

2. Semantic Variant (PPA-S)

Semantics is the study of meanings of word [108]. Severe progressive anomia is the hall mark of this variant which is a direct consequence of the loss of meanings of words [109].

Patients tend to ask the meanings of words repetitively [110] but lack insight of their impairment [99]. Speech fluency and repetition is preserved.

With progression of the semantic deficits, object recognition through sensory inputs other than speech is also impaired leading to inability to recognize smells (olfactory agnosia) [111], and inability to visually recognize objects (visual agnosia) [110] which may eventually lead to disturbance in facial recognition (progressive prosopagnosia) [112].

Imaging Characteristics

Selective atrophic changes affecting the anterior temporal lobes bilaterally, being more severe on the left, are characteristic of PPA-S [113-116].

Neuropathology

Most PPA-S cases have shown the histological picture of ubiquitinated frontotemporal lobar degeneration (FTLD-U) pathology with ubiquitin positive, tau-negative inclusions [117,118].

Associated Features

PPA-S has a strong association with the behavioral or frontal variant of Frontotemporal (bvFTD) [119, 120]. There is marked disinhibtion [121], increased social seeking [120] and extreme changes in food preferences [121] (the food fads [120]) leading at times to weight gain [121].

PPA-S may also be referred to as Semantic variant PPA (svPPA) [100], primary progressive semantic aphasia [122], fluent PPA [123], or temporal variant FrontoTemporal Dementia [124] and was originally named semantic dementia (SD) [125].

3. Logopenic Variant (PPA-L)

This is the most recently recognized variant of PPA [115] and displays some features of both the other variants [126]. Spontaneous speech is slow like

PPA-G but unlike it, is free from major agrammatic errors [95]. The naming impairment is less severe than PPA-S, and the meanings of words are not lost [95]. As suggested by preserved repetition of single words and impaired sentence repetition, short-term phonologic memory losses have been hypothesized to be the basic mechanism of aphasia in these patients [127].

Imaging Characteristics

Atrophic changes are seen in superior and middle temporal gyri posteriorly and in the inferior parietal lobule [115]. There have been recent reports of involvement of the left medial temporo-parietal cortex, right temporo-parietal cortex, and left inferior frontal cortex accompanied by corresponding white matter atrophy in these regions as well [127-129].

Neuropathology

PPA-L has been shown to be strongly associated with the Alzheimer's disease (AD) pathology [12].

Associated Features

Behavioral abnormalities like apathy, anxiety, and irritability may be seen [119, 129].

PPA-L may also be referred to as the Logopenic variant PPA (lvPPA) [91], Logopenic Progressive Aphasia (LPA) [115] or progressive mixed aphasia [14, 102, 130].

Treatment and Prognosis of PPA

The clinical utility of speech and language therapy has not been studied enough to warrant the formulation of standard guidelines for PPA, however, a beneficial role does seem probable [131]. Similarly the use of pharmaceutical agents is also only in the early stages of exploration [91], although Memantine has shown to be of potential benefit in the agrammatic variant (PPA-G) [132].

The established interventions include education, counseling and support for the patient and caregivers along with the medical amelioration of associated behavioral symptoms e.g. prescribing Selective Serotonin Reuptake Inhibitors (SSRI) for agitation and food-fads [91, 133].

There is an acute shortage of epidemiological data for PPA [134]. What we do know is that PPA demonstrates a slow yet steady progress in language deterioration [14] which might start out as any one of the three variants but gradually goes on to show a mixed picture with extensive overlap between variants [91]. This deterioration remains confined to the language domain in the initial years but this might be the case for up to ten years [12]. Patients survive for an average of eight to ten years after diagnosis [105, 135] almost invariably dying of other diseases of old age [136].

Conclusion

The Aphasias, both classic and progressive, continue to take an enormous toll on human health and functionality. Present research points to the number of potential cures which need to be studied on larger scale over longer periods of time for the development of cost-effective strategies in preventing and curing this debilitating condition. Any breakthrough in developing an effective treatment for one category of aphasia may well be beneficial for other types as well. The treatment, management and understanding of the disease pathophysiology of aphasia remain a challenge in the coming years.

References

[1]   Marshall R. S., Lazar R. M., Mohr J. P. Aphasia. *Medical update for psychiatrists.* 1998; 3(5):132-138.

[2]   Damasio A. R. Aphasia. *N. Engl. J. Med.* 1992; 326:531–539.

[3]   Goodglass H. and Kaplan E. *The assessment of aphasia and related disorders,* 2nd ed. Philadelphia: Lea and Febiger ; 1983.

[4]   Finger S., Roe D. Does gustave Dax deserve to be forgotten? The temporal lobe theory and other contributions of an overlooked figure in the history of language and cerebral dominance. *Brain and Language.* 1999; 69(1):16-30.

[5]   Burns M. S., Fahy J. Broca's area: rethinking classical concepts from a neuroscience perspective. *Top Stroke Rehabil.* 2010; 17(6):401-410.

[6]   McIntosh A. R. Towards a network theory of cognition. *Neural. Netw.* 2000; 13:861–870.

[7]   Mesulam M. M. Large-scale neurocognitive networks and distributed processing for attention, language, and memory. *Ann. Neurol.* 1990; 28:597–613.

[8]   Knecht S., Deppe M., Dräger B., Bobe L., Lohmann H., Ringelstein E., et al. *Language lateralization in healthy right handers.* Brain. 2000; 123:74-81.

[9]   Szaflarski J. P., Binder J. R., Possing E. T., McKiernan K. A., Ward B. D., Hammeke T. A. Language lateralization in left-handed and ambidextrous people: fMRI data. *Neurology.* 2002; 59(2):238.

[10]   Marien P., Engelborghs S., Vignolo L. A., De Deyn P. P. The many faces of crossed aphasia in dextrals: report of nine cases and review of the literature. *Eur. J. Neurol.* 2001; 8:643–58.

[11]   Ozyürek A., Kelly S. D. Gesture, brain, and language. *Brain Lang.* 2007; 101(3):181-4.

[12]   Mesulam M. Chapter 26. Aphasia, Memory Loss, and Other Focal Cerebral Disorders. In: Longo D. L., Fauci A. S., Kasper D. L., Hauser S. L., Jameson J. L., Loscalzo J., eds. *Harrison's Principles of Internal Medicine.* 18th ed. New York: McGraw-Hill; 2012.

[13]   Catani M., Ffytche D. H. The rises and falls of disconnection syndromes. *Brain.* 2005; 128(10):2224–2239.

[14]   Mesulam M., Wieneke C., Rogalski E., Cobia D., Thompson C. K., Weintraub S. Quantitative template for subtyping primary progressive aphasia. *Arch. Neurol.* 2009; 66:1545–1551.

[15]   Broca P. Perte de la parole. Romollisement chronique et destruction partielle du lobe anterieur gauche du cerveau. *Bull. Soc. Anthropol.* 1861;2.

[16]   Hillis A. E. Aphasia: progress in the last quarter of a century. *Neurology.* 2007; 69:200–213.

[17]   Fazio P., Cantagallo A., Craighero L., D'Ausilio A., Roy A. C., Pozzo T., Calzolari F., Granieri E., Fadiga L. Encoding of human action in Broca's area. *Brain.* 2009;132; 1980–1988.

[18]   Ropper A. H., Samuels M. A. Chapter 23. Disorders of Speech and Language. In: Ropper A. H., Samuels M. A., eds. *Adams and Victor's Principles of Neurology.* 9th ed. New York: McGraw-Hill; 2009.

[19]   Yang Z. H., Zhao X. Q., Wang C. X., Chen H. Y., Zhang Y. M. Neuroanatomic correlation of the post-stroke aphasias studied with imaging. *Neurol. Res.* 2008; 30(4): 356-360.

[20]   Mohr J. P., Pessin M. S., Finkelstein S., Funkenstein H. H., Duncan G. W., Davis K. R. Broca aphasia: pathologic and clinical. *Neurology.* 1978; 28(4):311-324.

[21] Ochfeld E., Newhart M., Molitoris J., et al. Ischemia in Broca area is associated with Broca aphasia more reliably in acute than in chronic stroke. *Stroke.* 2010; 41:325–330.

[22] Ardila A. A proposed reinterpretation and reclassification of aphasic syndromes. *Aphasiology.* 2010; 24(3):363-394.

[23] Gainotti G., Miceli G., Caltagirone C. Contiguity versus similarity paraphasic substitutions in Broca's and in Wernicke's aphasia. *J. Commun. Disord.* 1981; 14(1):1-9.

[24] Wernicke C. Der aphasiche symptomenkomplex:Eine psychologische studie auf anatomischer basis. Breslau: Cohn and Weigert, 1874.

[25] Goodglass H., Kaplan E. and Barresi B. *The assessment of aphasia and related disorders,* 3rd ed. Baltimore: Lippincott Williams andWilkins; 2001a.

[26] Kertesz A., Lau W. K., Polk M. The structural determinants of recovery in Wernicke's Aphasia. *Brain Lang.* 1993; 44:153–164.

[27] Hanlon R. E., Lux W. E., Dromerick A. W. Global aphasia without hemiparesis: language profiles and lesion distribution. *J. Neurol. Neurosurg. Psychiatry.* 1999; 66:365–369.

[28] Oliveira F. F., Damasceno B. P. Global aphasia as a predictor of mortality in the acute phase of a first stroke. *Arq. Neuropsiquiatr.* 2011; 69(2B):277-282.

[29] Lin J. H., Kwan S. Y., Wu D. Postictal aphasia with transient sulcal hyperintensity on M. R. I. *J. Chin. Med. Assoc.* 2006; 69(10):499-502.

[30] Lichtheim L. On aphasia. *Brain.* 1885; 7:443-484.

[31] Anderson J. M., Gilmore R., Roper S., Crosson B., Bauer R. M., Nadeau S., et al. Conduction aphasia and the arcuate fasciculus: A reexamination of the Wernicke-Geschwind model. *Brain Lang.* 1999; 70:1–12.

[32] Goodglass H. *Diagnosis of conduction aphasia.* In S. E. Kohn editor. Conduction aphasia, Hillsdale, N. J.: Lawrence Erlbaum Associates; 1992. pp. 39-49.

[33] Geschwind N. Disconnection syndromes in animals and man. *Brain.* 1965; 88: 237–294, 585–644.

[34] Turken A., Whitfield-Gabrieli S., Bammer R., Baldo J. V., Dronkers N. F., Gabrieli J. D. Cognitive processing speed and the structure of white matter pathways: Convergent evidence from normal variation and lesion studies. *Neuroimage.* 2008; 42,1032–1044.

[35]   Axer H., von Keyserlingk A. G., Berks G., von Keyserlingk D. G.
       Supra- and infrasylvian conduction aphasia. *Brain and Language.* 2001;
       76: 317–331.
[36]   Yarnell P. R. Crossed dextral aphasia: a clinical radiological correlation.
       Brain and language 1981; 12,128–139.
[37]   Mendez M. F., Benson D. F. Atypical conduction aphasia: a
       disconnection syndrome. *Archives of Neurology.* 1985; 42: 886–891.
[38]   Selnes O. A., van Zijl P., Barker P. B., Hillis A. E., Mori S.,
       M. R. diffusion tensor imaging documented arcuate fasciculus lesion
       in a patient with normal repetition performance. *Aphasiology.* 2002;
       16:897–902.
[39]   Rauschecker A. M., Deutsch G. K., Ben-Shachar M., Schwartzman A.,
       Perry L. M., Dougherty R. F. Reading impairment in a patient with
       missing arcuate fasciculus. *Neuropsychologia.* 2009; 47:180–194.
[40]   Goldstein K. Pictures of speech disturbances due to impairment of the
       non-language mental performances. In: *Language and language
       disturbances.* New-York: Grune and Stratton; 1948. pp. 292–309.
[41]   Geschwind N., Quadfasel F. A., Sagarra J. M. Isolation of the speech
       area. *Neuropsychologia.* 1968; 6(4):327–40.
[42]   Masdeu J. C., Schoene W. C., Funkenstein H. H. Aphasia following
       infarction of the left supplementary motor area. *Neurology.* 1979;
       15:627–653.
[43]   Freedman M., Alexander M. P., Naeser M. A. Anatomic basis of
       transcortical motor aphasia. *Neurology.* 1984; 34: 409–417.
[44]   Kumral E., Bayulkem G., Evyapan D., Yunten N. Spectrum of anterior
       cerebral artery territory infarction: clinical and M. R. I. findings. *Eur. J.
       Neurol.* 2002; 9(6):615-624.
[45]   Alexander M. P., Hiltbrunner B., Fischer R. S. Distributed anatomy of
       transcortical sensory aphasia. *Arch. Neurol.* 1989; 46:885–892.
[46]   Maeshima S., Toshiro H., Sekiguchi E., Okita R., Yamaga H., Ozaki F.,
       Moriwaki H., Matsumoto T., Ueyoshi A., Roger P. Transcortical mixed
       aphasia due to cerebral infarction in left inferior frontal lobe and
       temporo-parietal lobe. *Neuroradiology.* 2002; 44(2):133-137.
[47]   Andreetta S., Cantagallo A., Marini A. Narrative discourse in anomic
       aphasia. *Neuropsychologia.* 2012 May 5. [Epub ahead of print]
       P. M. I. D.: 22564448.
[48]   Okuda B., Kawabata K., Tachibana H., Sugita M., Tanaka H.
       Postencephalitic pure anomic aphasia: 2 year follow-up. *J. Neurol. Sci.*
       2001; 187:99–102.

[49] Miceli G., Giustolisi L., Caramazza A. The interaction of lexical and non-lexical processing mechanism: evidence from anomia. *Cortex.* 1991; 27:57–80.

[50] Yamawaki R., Suzuki K., Tanji K., Fujii T., Endo K., Meguro K., Yamadori A. Anomic alexia of kanji in a patient with anomic aphasia. *Cortex.* 2005 ; 41(4):555-559.

[51] Takeda M., Tachibana H., Shibuya N., Nakajima Y., Okuda B., Sugita M., Tanaka H. Pure anomic aphasia caused by a subcortical hemorrhage in the left temporo-parieto-occipital lobe. *Intern. Med.*1999; 38(3): 293-295.

[52] Hillis A. E., Wityk R. J., Barker P. B., Beauchamp H. J., Gailloud P., Murphy K., Cooper O., Metter E. J. Subcortical aphasia and neglect in acute stroke: the role of cortical hypoperfusion. *Brain.* 2002; 125(Pt 5):1094-1104.

[53] Damasio A. R., Damasio H., Rizzo M., Varney N., Gersh F. Aphasia with nonhemorrhagic lesions in the basal ganglia and internal capsule. *Arch Neurol.* 1982; 39:15–24.

[54] Cappa S. F., Cavallotti G., Guidotti M., Papagno C., Vignolo L. A. Subcortical aphasia: two clinical-CT scan correlation studies. *Cortex.* 1983; 19: 227–241.

[55] Alexander M. P., Naeser M. A., Palumbo C. L. Correlations of subcortical C. T. lesion sites and aphasia profiles. *Brain.* 1987; 110:961–991.

[56] de Boissezon X., Démonet J. F., Puel M., Marie N., Raboyeau G., Albucher J. F., Chollet F., Cardebat D. Subcortical aphasia: a longitudinal P. E. T. study. *Stroke. 2005;* 36(7):1467-1473.

[57] Hillis A. E., Barker A. E., Wityk R. J., Aldrich E. M., Restrepo L., Breese E. L., Work M. Variability in subcortical aphasia is due to variable sites of cortical hypoperfusion. *Brain Lang.* 2004; 89(3):524-530.

[58] Choi J. Y., Lee K. H., Na D. L., Byun H. S., Lee S. J., Kim H., Kwon M., Lee K.-H., Kim B.-T. Subcortical aphasia after striatocapsular infarction: quantitative analysis of brain perfusion S. P. E. C. T. using statistical parametric mapping and a statistical probabilistic anatomic map. *J. Nucl. Med.* 2007; 48: 194–200.

[59] Kauhanen M. L., Korpelainen J. T., Hiltunen P., Maatta R., Monoen H., Brusin E., et al. Aphasia, depression, and non-verbal cognitive impairment in ischaemic stroke. *Cerebrovasc. Dis.* 2000; 10: 455–461.

[60] Cobley C. S., Thomas S. A., Lincoln N. B., Walker M. F. The assessment of low mood in stroke patients with aphasia: reliability and validity of the 10-item Hospital version of the Stroke Aphasic Depression Questionnaire (SADQH-10). *Clin. Rehabil.* 2012; 26(4):372-381.

[61] Warlow C. P., Sandercock P., Dennis M. and Wardlaw J. *Stroke: a Practical Guide to Management.* Oxford: Blackwell Science; 2000.

[62] Pedersen P. M., Jorgensen H. S., Nakayama H., Raaschou H. O., Plsen T. S. Aphasia in acute stroke: incidence, determinants and recovery. *Ann. Neurol.* 1995; 38:659–666.

[63] Robey R. R. The efficacy of treatment for aphasic persons: a meta-analysis. *Brain Lang.* 1994; 47(4):582-608.

[64] Miniussi C. et al. Efficacy of repetitive transcranial magnetic stimulation/transcranial direct current stimulation in cognitive neurorehabilitation. *Brain Stimul.* 2008; 1: 326–336.

[65] Brady M. C., Kelly H., Godwin J., Enderby P. Speech and language therapy for aphasia following stroke. *Cochrane Database Syst. Rev.* 2012 May 16;5:CD000425.

[66] Aftonomos L. B., Appelbaum J. S., Steele R. D. Improving outcomes for persons with aphasia in advanced community-based treatment programs. *Stroke.* 1999; 30(7):1370-1379.

[67] Bhogal S. K., Teasell R., Speechley M. Intensity of aphasia therapy, impact on recovery. *Stroke.* 2003; 34(4):987-993.

[68] Fucetola R., Tucker F., Blank K., Corbetta M. A process for translating evidence-based aphasia treatment into clinical practice. *Aphasiology.* 2005; 19(3-5):411-422.

[69] Albert M. L. Treatment of aphasia. *Arch. Neurol.* 1998; 55(11):1417-1419.

[70] Kolk H., Heeschen C. Adaptation symptoms and impairment symptoms in Broca's aphasia. *Aphasiology*; 1990(4): 221–231.

[71] Berthier M. L., Pulvermüller F. Neuroscience insights improve neurorehabilitation of poststroke aphasia. *Nat. Rev. Neurol.* 2011; 7(2):86-97.

[72] Szaflarski J. P., Ball A., Grether S., Al-Fwaress F., Griffith N. M., Neils-Strunjas J., Newmeyer A., Reichhardt R. Constraint-induced aphasia therapy stimulates language recovery in patients with chronic aphasia after ischemic stroke. *Med. Sci. Monit.* 2008; 14(5):CR243-250.

[73] Cherney L. R., Patterson J. P., Raymer A., Frymark T., Schooling T. Evidence-based systematic review: effects of intensity of treatment and

constraint-induced language therapy for individuals with stroke-induced aphasia. *J. Speech Lang Hear Res.* 2008; 51(5):1282-1299.

[74] Meinzer M., Djundja D., Barthel G., Elbert T., Rockstroh B. Long-term stability of improved language functions in chronic aphasia after constraint-induced aphasia therapy. *Stroke.* 2005; 36(7):1462-1466.

[75] Small S. L., Llano D. A. Biological approaches to aphasia treatment. *Curr. Neurol. Neurosci.* 2009; 9(6): 443–450.

[76] Greener J., Enderby P., Whurr R. Pharmacological treatment for aphasia following stroke. *Cochrane Database Syst. Rev.* 2001;(4):CD000424.

[77] Winblad B. Piracetam: a review of pharmacological properties and clinical uses. *C. N. S. Drug Rev.* 2005; 11:169–182.

[78] Berthier M. L. Poststroke aphasia: epidemiology, pathophysiology and treatment. *Drugs Aging.* 2005; 22(2): 163–182.

[79] Berthier M. L., et al. Memantine and constraint induced aphasia therapy in chronic poststroke aphasia. *Ann. Neurol.* 2009; 65: 577–585.

[80] Wade D. T., Hewer R. L., David R. M., Enderby P. Aphasia after stroke: natural history and associated deficits. *J. Neurol. Neurosurg. Psychiatry.* 1986; 49:11–16.

[81] Draper B., Bowring G., Thompson C., Van Heyst J., Conroy P., Thompson J. Stress in caregivers of aphasic stroke patients: a randomized controlled trial. *Clin. Rehabil.* 2007; 21(2):122-130.

[82] Pedersen P. M., Jørgensen H. S., Nakayama H., Raaschou H. O., Olsen T. S. Aphasia in acute stroke: incidence, determinants, and recovery. *Ann. Neurol.* 1995; 38(4):659–666.

[83] Heiss W. D., Thiel A., Kessler J., et al. Disturbance and recovery of language function: correlates in P. E. T. activation studies. *Neuroimage* 2003;20(Suppl. 1):S42–49.

[84] Demeurisse G., Demol O., Derouck M., et al. Quantitative study of the rate of recovery from aphasia due to ischemic stroke. *Stroke.* 1980; 11:455–458.

[85] Farrell R., Evans S., Corbett D. Environmental enrichment enhances recovery of function but exacerbates ischemic cell death. *Neuroscience.* 2001; 107(4),585–592.

[86] Cramer S. C., Chopp M. Recovery recapitulates ontogeny. *Trends in Neuroscience.* 2000; 23(6): 265–271.

[87] Jones T. A., Schallert T. Overgrowth and pruning of dendrites in adult rats recovering from neocortical damage. *Brain Research.* 1992; 581(1): 156–160.

[88] Lendrem W., Lincoln N. B. Spontaneous recovery of language in patients with aphasia between 4 and 34 weeks after stroke. *J. Neurol. Neurosurg. Psychiatry.* 1985; 48:743–748.

[89] Mark V. W., Thomas B. E., Berndt R. S. Factors associated with improvements in global aphasia. *Aphasiology.* 1992; 6:121–134.

[90] Kertesz A. What do we learn from recovery from aphasia? *Adv. Neurol.* 1988; 47:277–292.

[91] Harciarek M., Kertesz A. Primary progressive aphasias and their contribution to the contemporary knowledge about the brain-language relationship. *Neuropsychol. Rev.* 2011 ; 21(3):271-287.

[92] Hodges J. R., Patterson K. Semantic dementia: a unique clinicopathological syndrome. *Lancet Neurology.* 2007; 6: 1004–1014.

[93] Sourdet S., Rougé-Bugat M. E., Vellas B., Forette F. Editorial: frailty and aging. *J. Nutr. Health Aging* 2012;16(4):283-284.

[94] Wiener J. M., Tilly J. Population ageing in the United States of America: implications for public programmes. *Int. J. Epidemiol.* 2002; 31:776–781.

[95] Gorno-Tempini M. L., Hillis A. E., Weintraub S., Kertesz A., Mendez M., Cappa S. F., Ogar J. M., Rohrer J. D., Black S., Boeve B. F., et al. Classification of primary progressive aphasia and its variants. *Neurology.* 2011; 76: 1006–1014.

[96] Knibb, J. A., Woollams, A. M., Hodges, J. R., and Patterson, K. (2009). Making sense of progressive non-fluent aphasia: an analysis of conversational speech. *Brain,* 132, 2734–2746.

[97] Ash S., Moore P., Veseley L., Gunawardena D., McMillan C., Anderson C., et al. Non-fluent speech in frontotemporal lobar degeneration. *Journal of Neurolinguistics.* 2009; 22: 370–383.

[98] Karbe H., Kertesz A., Polk M. Profiles of language impairment in primary progressive aphasia. *Archives of Neurology.* 1993; 50:193–201.

[99] Kertesz A. Anosognosia for aphasia. In G. P. Prigatano editor. *The study of anosognosia.* New York: Oxford University Press; 2010.

[100] Whitwell J. L., Avula R., Senjem M. L., Kantarci K., Weigand S. D., Samikoglu A., et al. Gray and white matter water diffusion in the syndromic variants of frontotemporal dementia. *Neurology.* 2010; 74: 1279–1287.

[101] Cappa S. F., Perani D., Messa C., Miozzo A., Fazio F. Varieties of progressive non-fluent aphasia. *Annals of the New York Academy of Science.* 1996; 777: 243–248.

[102] Mesulam M., Wicklund A., Johnson N., Rogalski E., Leger G. C., Rademaker A., et al. Alzheimer and frontotemporal pathology in subsets of primary progressive aphasia. *Annals of Neurology*. 2008; 63:709–719.

[103] Davies R. R. and Xuereb J. H. The histopathology of frontotemporal dementia. In J. R. Hodges editor. *Frontotemporal dementia syndromes*. New York: Cambridge University Press; 2007.

[104] Rohrer J. D., Paviour D., Bronstein A. M., O'Sullivan S. S., Lees A., Warren J. D. Progressive supranuclear palsy syndrome presenting as progressive nonfluent aphasia: a neuropsychological and neuroimaging analysis. *Movement Disorders*. 2010; 25: 179–188.

[105] Kertesz A., Blair M., McMonagle P., Munoz D. The diagnosis and course of frontotemporal dementia. *Alzheimer Disease and Associated Disorders*. 2007; 21: 155–163.

[106] Fukui T., Sugita K., Kawamura M., Shiota J., Nakano I. Primary progressive apraxia in Pick's disease: a clinicopathologic study. *Neurology*. 1996; 47:467–473.

[107] Grossman M., Mickanin J., Onishi K., Hughes E., D'Esposito M., Ding X. S., et al. Progressive non-fluent aphasia: Language, cognitive and PET measures contrasted with probable Alzheimer's disease. *Journal of Cognitive Neuroscience*. 1996; 8:135– 154.

[108] Taber's Cyclopedic Medical Dictionary. 20th ed. Philadelphia: F. A. Davis Company; 2005. *Semantics*; p.1969.

[109] Harciarek M., Kertesz A. Longitudinal study of singleword comprehension in semantic dementia: a comparison with primary progressive aphasia and Alzheimer's disease. *Aphasiology*. 2009; 23: 606–626.

[110] Kertesz A., Jesso S., Harciarek M., Blair M., McMonagle, P. What is semantic dementia?: a cohort study of diagnostic features and clinical boundaries. *Archives of Neurology*. 2010; 67: 483– 489.

[111] Luzzi S., Snowden J. S., Neary D., Coccia M., Provinciali L., Lambon Ralph M. A. Distinct patterns of olfactory impairment in Alzheimer's disease, semantic dementia, frontotemporal dementia, and corticobasal degeneration. *Neuropsychologia*. 2007; 45:1823–1831.

[112] Josephs K. A., Whitwell J. L., Vemuri P., Senjem M. L., Boeve B. F., Knopman D. S., et al. The anatomic correlate of prosopagnosia in semantic dementia. *Neurology*. 2008; 71: 1628– 1633.

[113] Hodges J. R., Patterson K., Oxbury S., Funnell E. Semantic dementia. Progressive fluent aphasia with temporal lobe atrophy. *Brain*. 1992; 115: 1783–1806.

[114] Galton C. J., Patterson K., Graham K., Lambon-Ralph M. A., Williams G., Antoun N., et al. Differing patterns of temporal atrophy in Alzheimer's disease and semantic dementia. *Neurology*. 2001; 57: 216–225.

[115] Gorno-Tempini M. L., Dronkers N. F., Rankin K. P., Ogar J. M., Phengrasamy L., Rosen H. J., et al. Cognition and anatomy in three variants of primary progressive aphasia. *Annals of Neurology*. 2004; 55: 335–346.

[116] Rosen H. J., Gorno-Tempini M. L., Goldman W. P., Perry R. J., Schuff N., Weiner M., et al. Patterns of brain atrophy in frontotemporal dementia and semantic dementia. *Neurology*. 2002; 58:198–208.

[117] Davies R. R., Hodges J. R., Kril J. J., Patterson K., Halliday G. M., Xuereb J. H. The pathological basis of semantic dementia. *Brain*. 2005; 128:1984–1995.

[118] Kertesz A., McMonagle P., Blair M., Davidson W., Munoz D. G. The evolution and pathology of frontotemporal dementia. *Brain*. 2005;128: 1996–2005.

[119] Rosen H. J., Allison S. C., Ogar J. M., Amici S., Rose K., Dronkers N., et al. Behavioral features in semantic dementia vs other forms of progressive aphasias. *Neurology*. 2006;67:1752–1756.

[120] Snowden J. S., Bathgate D., Varma A., Blackshaw A., Gibbons Z. C., Neary D. Distinct behavioural profiles in frontotemporal dementia and semantic dementia. *Journal of Neurology, Neurosurgery, and Psychiatry*. 2001; 70:323–332.

[121] Seeley W. W., Bauer A. M., Miller B. L., Gorno-Tempini M. L., Kramer J. H., Weiner M., et al. The natural history of temporal variant frontotemporal dementia. *Neurology*. 2005; 64:1384–1390.

[122] Kertesz A., Davidson W., McCabe P. Primary progressive semantic aphasia: a case study. *Journal of the International Neuropsychological Society*. 1998; 4:388–398.

[123] Adlam A. L., Patterson K., Rogers T. T., Nestor P. J., Salmond C. H., Acosta-Cabronero J., et al. Semantic dementia and fluent primary progressive aphasia: two sides of the same coin? *Brain*. 2006; 129:3066–3080.

[124] Bozeat S., Gregory C. A., Ralph M. A., Hodges J. R. Which neuropsychiatric and behavioural features distinguish frontal and temporal variants of frontotemporal dementia from Alzheimer's disease? *Journal of Neurology, Neurosurgery, and Psychiatry*. 2000; 69: 178–186.

[125] Snowden J. S., Goulding P. J., Neary D. Semantic dementia: a form of circumscribed cerebral atrophy. *Behavioural Neurology.* 1989; 2:167–182.

[126] Etcheverry L., Seidel B., Grande M., Schulte S., Pieperhoff P., Südmeyer M., Minnerop M., Binkofski F., Huber W., Grodzinsky Y., Amunts K., Heim S. The time course of neurolinguistic and neuropsychological symptoms in three cases of logopenic primary progressive aphasia. *Neuropsychologia.* 2012; 50(7):1708-1718.

[127] Gorno-Tempini M. L., Brambati S. M., Ginex V., et al. The logopenic/phonological variant of primary progressive aphasia. *Neurology.* 2008; 71:1227–1234.

[128] Migliaccio R., Agosta F., Rascovsky K., Karydas A., Bonasera S., Rabinovici G. D., et al. Clinical syndromes associated with posterior atrophy: early age at onset A. D. spectrum. *Neurology.* 2009; 73:1571–1578.

[129] Rohrer J. D., Warren J. D. Phenomenology and anatomy of abnormal behaviours in primary progressive aphasia. *Journal of the Neurological Sciences.* 2010; 29:35–38.

[130] Grossman M. Primary progressive aphasia: clinicopathological correlations. Nature Review. *Neurology.* 2010; 6:88–97.

[131] Henry M. L., Beeson P. M., Rapcsak S. Z. Treatment for lexical retrieval in progressive aphasia. *Aphasiology.* 2008; 22(7-8):826-838.

[132] Boxer A. L., Lipton A. M., Womack K., Merrilees J., Neuhaus J., Pavlic D., et al. An open-label study of Memantine treatment in 3 subtypes of frontotemporal lobar degeneration. *Alzheimer Disease and Associated Disorders,* 2009; 23:211–217.

[133] Lebert F., Stekke W., Hasenbroekx C., Pasquier F. Frontotemporal dementia: a randomised, controlled trial with trazodone. *Dementia and Geriatric Cognitive Disorders,* 2004; 17:355–359.

[134] Code C., Petheram B. Delivering for aphasia. *Int. J. Speech Lang Pathol.* 2011; 13(1):3-10.

[135] Hodges J. R., Davies R., Xuereb J., Kril J., Halliday G. Survival in frontotemporal dementia. *Neurology.* 2003; 61:349–354.

[136] Gorina Y., Hoyert D., Lentzner H., Goulding M. Trends in causes of death among older persons in the United States. *Aging Trends,* No 6. Hyattsville, Maryland: National Center for Health Statistics. 2006.

[137] Sardar M. R., Kuntz C., Mazurek J. A., Akhtar N. H., Saeed W., Shapiro T. Recurrent takotsubo cardiomyopathy in the setting of transient

neurological symptoms: a case report. *J. Med. Case Rep.* 2011 Aug. 24;5:412.

Reviewer:

Eric Gnall, DO, Marwan Badri, MBChB and Adeel Siddiqui, MD. G10, Annenberg Education Center. 100 Lancaster Ave, Wynnewood P. A. 19096. Tel: 718-213-9554. E-mail: gnalle@mlhs.org, badrim@mlhs.org and SiddiquiAd@mlhs.org.

In: Aphasia   ISBN: 978-1-62257-681-4
Editors: E. Holmgren, E.S. Rudkilde © 2013 Nova Science Publishers, Inc.

Chapter III

Intensive Treatment, Pharmacotherapy, Transcranial Magnetic/electric Stimulation as Potential Adjuvant Treatment for Aphasia

Beatrice Leemann[1], and Marina Laganaro[2]*
[1]University Hospital of Geneva, Geneva, Switzerland
[2]University of Geneva, Geneva, Switzerland

Abstract

Aphasia after stroke is a common and disabling symptom, which can recover in the weeks, months or years following brain injury, showing that the adult brain can reorganize to adjust to impaired functions. Standard rehabilitation approaches aim to improve the deficient function through speech and language therapy (SLT). In parallel with increasing knowledge about central nervous system plasticity, different adjuvant interventions have been recently implemented to enhance the outcome of speech and language therapy. One of them consists in increasing the intensity of SLT in order to obtain better recovery. This is achieved for

* Tél. +41(22) 37 23 614; Fax +41(22) 37 23 644; beatrice.leemann@hcuge.ch.

instance with computer-assisted therapy (CAT) or with constraint-induced aphasia therapy (CIAT) approaches.

A second approach tested the combination of a number of drugs with SLT, with the aim to increase its effect. The mechanism thought to underlie enhanced recovery with the addition of specific drugs includes increasing attention and learning though modulation of neurotransmission or restoring metabolic function. Several substances have been assessed, including noradrenergic drugs and drugs acting on the dopaminergic, glutaminergic, gabaergic, and cholinergic systems.

Finally, another, still experimental, intervention in stroke rehabilitation consists of neuromodulation via non-invasive cortical stimulation, e.g. through transcranial magnetic stimulation (TMS) or direct current stimulation (tDCS). These techniques have recently been proposed to potentially endorse functional recovery after stroke through (i) enhancing excitability of the stroke hemisphere or (ii) suppressing the non-stroke hemisphere to reduce its potential interference with functional recovery of the stroke hemisphere.

While both treatment intensity and TMS have led to several promising results on efficacy in aphasia rehabilitation, the effect of pharmacotherapy seems to be less straightforward. In the present chapter we will perform a review of recent literature on the effects of these approaches as potential adjuvant to standard SLT in the rehabilitation of aphasia.

Acronyms

AAT	Aachen aphasia test
CAT	computer-assisted therapy
CIAT	constraint-induced aphasia therapy
CILT	constraint-induced language therapy
NMDA	N-methyl-D-aspartate
PICA	Porch index of communication ability
RCT	randomized controlled trial
SLT	speech and language therapy
rTMS	repetitive transcranial magnetic stimulation
tDCS	transcranial direct current stimulation
WAB-AQ	Western aphasia battery- aphasia quotient

Introduction

Aphasia can occur in association with a wide range of brain injury and represents a common severe cognitive consequence following stroke as incidence of aphasia in stroke patients has been estimated around 30% (Engelter, Gostynski et al. 2006).

Spontaneous recovery can be expected in the acute phase by reperfusion of partially damaged tissue, resolution of edema, then resolution of diaschisis. In the sub-acute phase, reorganization within undamaged areas has been observed both in perilesional tissues in the left hemisphere and homologue areas in the right hemisphere (Saur and Hartwigsen 2012).

Speech and language therapy (SLT) is a generally accepted treatment modality for aphasia following stroke (Cicerone, Dahlberg et al. 2005). Rehabilitation training with SLT aims to achieve functional reorganization through plasticity in view to enhance functional outcome. However, efficacy and outcome of SLT are not always optimal (Kelly, Brady et al. 2010). That's why research still needs to address which conditions allow to optimize SLT and its outcome. In the present chapter we will briefly review SLT conditions known to optimize its efficacy, in particular treatment intensity, before describing an overview of some very different potential adjuvant to SLT, namely computer assisted treatment, pharmacotherapy and transcranial magnetic or electric stimulation.

Learning and Plasticity

As a matter of fact neural plasticity that supports learning in healthy subjects is also the adaptive mechanism which allows reorganization to restore or compensate lost functions ("relearning").

Neural plasticity includes molecular modifications (e.g. changes in gene expression), cellular modifications (for example dendritic growth), synaptic modification (synaptogenesis, increased synaptic responses, long term potentiation), circuit modification with reorganization of representation (cortical map reorganization) and finally change in activation patterns-neural connectivity (Raymer, Beeson et al. 2008), (Kleim and Jones 2008).

Acknowledging the diversity of these underlying processes is important because of their direct implication in rehabilitation. We will briefly mention a few of them.

- Lack of activation of specific neuronal circuits leads to synaptic weaknesses and it constitutes the basis of the "learned non use". The typical example is a patient with arm paresis who avoids using it, preferring the unaffected arm. A specific intervention has been suggested to avoid "learned non use" in the motor domain, namely "constraint induce therapy", first developed by Taub and colleagues (Taub, Uswatte et al. 1999) which consists of restraining the unaffected limb to limit its use and a training program for the affected limb. Similarly, a patient with aphasia might avoid verbal communication, replacing it with gestures and pointing or restricting verbal communication to a limited set of utterances. The aim of this kind of intervention in the language domain would be therefore to force the patient to use all his residual language skills (constraint induced aphasia therapy (CIAT), (Pulvermuller, Neininger et al. 2001).

- It is arguable that treatment focused on one particular aspect of language would have a different result according to the SLT approach (Thompson 2000). The lack of generalization to untreated items (treatment specificity) has been shown in various treatment studies and in particular in anomia studies, where the improvement in naming is restricted to the treated items (Laganaro, Di Pietro et al. 2006). The number and the choice of treated items are therefore important.

- There is some evidence that action and perception systems co activate with the language system. For example reading action verbs activated a somatotopic pattern within premotor and motor cortex (Hauk, Johnsrude et al. 2004). Because of this interaction, relevant context may possibly facilitate language processes (Pulvermuller and Berthier 2008).

- Salience is important: the more the stimulus has salient "weight" for the subjects (for example in animal model stimuli allowing reception of a reward), the easier it is encoded. The basal forebrain cholinergic system probably contributes to saliency (Kleim and Jones 2008) and cortical plasticity (Conner, Chiba et al. 2005) and has lead to the introduction of pharmacological treatment based on anti cholinesterase drugs. Moreover, dopamine, seems to mediate the incentive salience of a reward and plays a role in motivation (Berridge and Robinson 1998).

- Finally learning is driven by correlation. The more frequently a neuronal circuit is activated in a synchronous manner, greater the synaptic strengths. The importance of intense (quantity) and high frequency treatment for aphasia is derived from these underlying learning processes (Berthier and Pulvermuller 2011) and it is discussed below.

In sum, a series of neurobiological mechanisms contribute to brain plasticity and relearning. Efficient SLT may rely on some of them more specifically; alternatively, some adjuvant treatments may improve the effects of SLT by priming or optimizing the underlying neurobiological mechanisms.

Treatment Intensity

As mentioned above, based on the way repetition strengthens synapses, treatment intensity seems to have a critical impact on recovery.

As a matter of fact in a meta analysis including published research between 1975-2002 (Bhogal, Teasell et al. 2003), the authors concluded on no effect of SLT in studies in which 2 hours weekly sessions of SLT were provided over a period of 22, 9 weeks, whereas significant effects of SLT were observed when an average of 8,8 hours of weekly therapy was provided over 11, 2 weeks. Not only the total number of therapy hours but also the number of weekly sessions ("massed practice") was significantly correlated to greater improvement on language assessment tests (Bhogal, Teasell et al. 2003). A systematic review of the Cochrane group including 30 trials between 1966 to April 2009 also found consistent evidence in favor of effectiveness of intensive SLT (Kelly, Brady et al. 2010), although Cherney and colleagues make more cautious conclusions in an another systematic review (Cherney, Patterson et al. 2011).

Furthermore, treatment intensity can be modulated not only by increasing the total number of SLT session but also in terms of number of treated items and item repetition (drill) during therapy and finally in terms of massed practice, namely sessions grouped over a short period rather than distributed over a longer time period. Increasing SLT intensity is not always possible due to a series of limitations in the health-care system (manly due to costs), but there are a few alternative/adjuvant ways to increase treatment intensity. Among these methods constraint-induced aphasia therapy (CIAT) and computer-assisted therapy (CAT) will be presented in the following section.

Constraint-Induced Aphasia Therapy

In constraint-induced aphasia therapy (CIAT) (Pulvermuller, Neininger et al. 2001) intense massed practice is combine with forced verbal language use. It consists of a therapeutic game activity carried out in small groups of aphasic patients with a therapist. The "game" is played with a set of cards with pictures on it, including two identical copies of each card. The task is to explicitly request the second card from another player. All requests have to be performed with verbal language. Shaping is performed by new explicit rules including the requirement to use the name of the co-players, politeness formulas, determiners, and so on.

In a randomized controlled trial Pulvermüller et al. compared two groups of chronic aphasic patients with the same amount of treatment but either massed over 10 days of 3 hour sessions of CIAT, or 4 week of conventional therapy. Significant improvement on 3 different clinical tests (naming, comprehension, Token test scores) was reported in the CIAT group and limited improvement in the control group. In addition, improvement in everyday communication was only observed in the CIAT group, (Pulvermuller, Neininger et al. 2001).

Further studies replicated the efficacy of CIAT (30 hours of training over 10 days) to improve language function in a larger sample of chronic aphasic patient (27) and results were stable at a 6 month follow up assessment (Meinzer, Djundja et al. 2005).

Maher and colleagues compared constraint-induced language therapy (CILT) defined as limiting the response only to spoken verbal production with promoting aphasic communicative effectiveness (PACE) therapy allowing all modes of communication, in a dual card game. Both groups received the same amount of therapy (3 hours, 4 days a week during 2 weeks) but they were not randomized. Positive results were observed in both groups but there was more consistent improvement in the CILT group on standard measures and on some aspects of narrative discourse (Maher, Kendall et al. 2006) showing that intensity is not the only important factor.

In a review of 10 studies (Cherney, Patterson et al. 2008) and in a recent review (Meinzer, Rodriguez et al. 2012) the authors conclude that there is indeed evidence of beneficial effects of CIAT on language functions. However, the reviews also outlined that the relative contribution of each of the aspects of CIAT (particularly massed practice and constraint verbal use) need to be further investigated (Meinzer, Rodriguez et al. 2012). Other studies concluded to limited effects of CIAT which were not maintained 3 months after treatment (Faroqi-Shah and Virion 2009).

Computer Assisted Therapy

An alternative way of increasing treatment intensity is implementing computer assisted therapy (CAT). CAT has several practical advantages for SLT, ranging from the possibility of increasing treatment intensity in terms of number of sessions and drill to a larger involvement of patient in therapy with increased autonomy and the possibility of controlling several parameters of stimuli presentation and feed-back.

CAT has been introduced since the 1980s in aphasia treatment, but a first review published in 1990 concluded that these first attempts did not prove its efficacy (Robertson 1990). In later years an increased number of studies have investigated the efficacy of CAT. As for other SLT approaches, most CAT studies targeted anomia treatment in aphasic patients (Fink, Brecher et al. 2002), (Laganaro, Di Pietro et al. 2003), (Pedersen, Vinter et al. 2001) and a few of them targeted other domains such as sentence comprehension (Crerar, Ellis et al. 1996), agraphia (Mortley, Enderby et al. 2001) and alexia (Laganaro and Overton Venet 2001). As a consequence, a second review on CAT published in 2004 concluded that several studies have proved the efficacy of CAT when specific linguistic domains are targeted (Wertz and Katz 2004). CAT studies have been shown to improve recovery from aphasia in chronic patients, but also in studies carried out with patients in the post-acute stage. In the latter studies, CAT sessions have been added to standard SLT sessions (Laganaro, Di Pietro et al. 2006). As a consequence, CAT allowed increasing treatment intensity from one to two daily sessions. Alternatively, CAT can also be delivered at home (Mortley, Wade et al. 2004), also allowing high intensity treatment. As an example, in a single patient study by Laganaro and Overton (2003), the patient worked at home daily on average 70 minutes during 3 weeks on a CAT for alexia. Finally, CAT enables intensity in terms of increased item-repetition (drill), which is also an essential condition for (re-)learning (see above). In a study on CAT for anomia, each of the 8 patients who received CAT with the same program repeated each item the number of times they estimated necessary, which varied from 5 to 21 times (Laganaro, Di Pietro et al. 2006a); in another study including patients presenting with similar anomia severity at baseline, each of the 3 patients achieved 85% of accuracy after a number of sessions varying from simple to double (Laganaro, Di Pietro et al. 2006b). These two examples illustrate how CAT also enables the adaptation of treatment intensity in terms of drill and of number of sessions for individual patients.

Pharmacological Treatment

Rationale for pharmacological treatment of aphasia is based mostly on two purposes: strengthing neural activity in networks mediating attention, word learning and memory and reestablishing the activity of neurotransmitters in dysfunctional brain region (Berthier, Pulvermuller et al. 2011).

Several substances have been assessed in studies with aphasic patients, including drugs acting on the noradrenergic, dopaminergic, glutaminergic, gabaergic, cholinergic systems. We will briefly review each of these groups of drugs.

Noradrenergic

D-amphetamine (or Dexamphetamine or Dextroamphetamine)

D-amphetamine acts mainly on the noradrenergic and dopaminergic systems and therefore possibly increases general brain excitability. After experimental infarction in rats it enhances neurite growth and synaptogenesis (Stroemer, Kent et al. 1998). Several studies have been published about the effect of amphetamine in combination with physiotherapy in motor recovery with a trend towards greater improvement in the amphetamine group (Sonde and Lokk 2007).

D-amphetamine has been found to enhance language learning in healthy subjects (Breitenstein, Wailke et al. 2004), (Whiting, Chenery et al. 2008). D-amphetamine has also been explored to favor recovery in aphasic patients. A double-blind placebo controlled study has been carried out with 21 stroke aphasic patients in the post-acute stage receiving 10 mg of dextroamphetamine or placebo, 30 min before speech therapy during 5 weeks. The authors reported that amphetamine paired with speech therapy accelerated immediate recovery from aphasia, on the Porch Index Communication Ability (PICA), but at 6 months no significant difference was found between the two groups (Walker-Batson, Curtis et al. 2001).

A smaller placebo-controlled, crossover design, shows that 2 chronic aphasic patients correctly named treated items more accurately under amphetamine than under placebo but the gain was statistically significant in only one patient (Whiting, Chenery et al. 2007).

However in clinical practice the administration of amphetamines is limited by the potentially serious side effects notably on blood pressure (Martinsson, Hardemark et al. 2007).

Dopaminergic

Dopamine contributes to synaptic plasticity (including long term potentiation) in different brain areas (hippocampus, striatum and prefrontal cortex) and seems to be a regulator in synaptic changes observed in learning and memory (Jay 2003). Different substances can act on the dopaminergic system, including levodopa (dopaminergic precursor), bromocriptine (dopaminergic agonist), moclobemide (monoamine oxydase inhibitor), and amantadine (dopamine releaser).

Levodopa

Some studies have shown an effect of levodopa on motor learning in young healthy volunteers and elderly subject (Floel, Breitenstein et al. 2005) and in patients following a stroke (Rosser, Heuschmann et al. 2008), (Scheidtmann, Fries et al. 2001). For instance, Levodopa as compared to placebo accelerated and improved word learning in 40 healthy subjects (Knecht, Breitenstein et al. 2004).

In aphasic patients, two randomized double blind placebo-controlled studies reported contradictory results in the acute phase, using similar doses of levodopa (100 mg) during 3 and respectively 2 weeks. In one study with 19 subjects, larger improvement was observed in the patients receiving levodopa than in the placebo group in three subtests of the Boston diagnostic aphasia examination: animal naming (verbal fluency), sentences and words repetition (Seniow, Litwin et al. 2009). By contrast in the other study, involving 12 patients, levodopa did not modulate the amount of improvement obtain with therapy (CAT) (Leemann, Laganaro et al. 2011).

In conclusion the potential effect of levodopa on recovery from aphasia remains controversial, even if it is postulated that disruption of dopamine pathways may play a role in distinctive features of non fluent aphasia (Berthier 2005).

Bromocriptine

A few single and multiple case reports and open label trials using bromocriptine reported improvement in language performance in non fluent chronic aphasic patients: 1 patient increased his naming accuracy and then returned to baseline after discontinuation (Albert, Bachman et al. 1988), 3 out of 7 patients (those with moderate aphasia) showed significant improvement on a lexical index and verbal fluency task, but also only the time the drug was given, (Sabe, Leiguarda et al. 1992), and 4 patients experienced significant increase in word retrieval, followed by a decrease after withdraw (Gold, VanDam et al. 2000).

In a randomized double blind placebo-controlled study on chronic non fluent aphasic patients, bromocriptine combined with SLT improved in particular verbal latency, reading comprehension, and qualitative measures of spontaneous speech in 5 patients (Bragoni, Altieri et al. 2000). The principal limitation of this study is that many patients were excluded during the recruitment phase (14 out of 25) and there was also a high rate of dropouts (6 of 11) due to secondary effects. Here again the effect on verbal latency was not sustained after wash-out.

Efficacy of bromocriptine in non fluent aphasia was not confirmed in one open label trial (Ozeren, Sarica et al. 1995) and in three randomized double blind placebo-controlled study, as well in the acute phase on 38 patients with maximal dose 10 mg /day (Ashtary, Janghorbani et al. 2006) as in studies carried out in the chronic phase with different doses (Gupta, Mlcoch et al. 1995) (Sabe, Leiguarda et al. 1992). Nevertheless the major limitation of these last two studies is that no SLT was given during the trial period.

In summary bromocriptine in chronic non fluent aphasia, associated with SLT, has a possibly, but not lasting, effect on verbal latencies.

Moclobemide

No difference between moclobemide (daily for 6 months) and placebo has been reported with a large (90 patients) double blind, placebo randomized study, with patients in the acute stage (Laska, von Arbin et al. 2005).

Amantadine

Amantadine increases the release of dopamine and norepinephrine but has also anti cholinergic proprieties and week antagonism of NMDA receptor (Berthier, Pulvermuller et al. 2011). An open label trial in 4 transcortical motor aphasic patients, using multiple assessments during on –off drug periods suggested that amantadine paired with SLT improves performance in a word generation task (Barrett and Eslinger 2007).

Piracetam (Pyrrolidone Acetamide)

Research on piracetam showed an effect in a variety of neurological disorders with some effects on memory, attention, cognition and depression (Malykh and Sadaie 2010).

The exact mechanism by which piracetam acts to improve these functions is unknown because piracetam is a non-specific pharmacological agent which seems to have a role in energy metabolism, particularly through its effect on cell membrane, a gaba-mimetic action, and its activation of AMPA-type glutamate receptors (Malykh and Sadaie 2010). It enhances also neurotransmission of acetylcholine (Huber 1999),(Berthier and Pulvermuller 2011).

They are many studies using piracetam in the acute phase after stroke including several studies on aphasia. Enderby et al performed a 12 week, double blind, parallel randomized placebo-controlled study with 158 post stoke patients, including 67 with aphasia. Patients also received SLT although its type and intensity was not mentioned. Higher improvement was reported for the piracetam group relative to the placebo group on several language assessment tests, but these benefits were not maintained 24 weeks later (Enderby, Broeckx et al. 1994).

A very large (N=927 stroke patients) multicenter RCT including a subgroup of aphasic patients evaluated the effectiveness of piracetam provided early after stroke during 12 weeks (De Deyn, De Reuck et al. 1997). Recovery from aphasia was particularly high in the group of patient treated within 7 hours post onset (Orgogozo 1999),(Huber 1999). However aphasia was not investigated in details but only documented with screening tests.

In a RCT including 66 aphasic patients, piracetam or placebo was associated with SLT during a 6-week period. In the piracetam group a significant effect was reported on the written language subtest of the Aachen aphasia test (AAT) (Huber, Willmes et al. 1997).

In another RCT study involving 24 aphasic patients within 14 days post stroke, piracetam or placebo were also given for 6 weeks in conjunction with SLT. Both groups displayed some improvement in token test, AAT subtest for written language and comprehension but the piracetam group also showed significant improvement in spontaneous speech (Kessler, Thiel et al. 2000).

On the other hand there was no clear beneficial effect of piracetam in a RCT of 49 aphasic patients receiving 4800 mg of piracetam or placebo during 6 months. However, there was no intensive SLT associated to pharmacotherapy in this study and only 30 of the 49 patients were finally analyzed (Gungor, Terzi et al. 2011).

In sum, piracetam seems to be an effective treatment of aphasia in combination with SLT when given in the acute phase post stroke and has a low incidence of mild adverse events (Noble and Benfield 1998).

Glutaminergic

Glutaminergic over activation of N methyl D aspartate (NMDA) receptors results in intercellular calcium overload, causing some neuronal dysfunction and death. Therefore one of the rational to use N methyl D aspartate (NMDA) glutamate receptor antagonist is the expected neuroprotective effect. Memantine, a NMDA receptor antagonist versus placebo has been investigated in a RCT with 27 chronic post stroke aphasic patients. The memantine group displayed higher improvement than the placebo group and recovery was even greater when speech therapy CIAT was added (Berthier, Green et al. 2009).

On the other hand, recently it has been demonstrated that hyper activation of NMDA is then followed by prolonged decrease in NMDA function. Thus perhaps stimulation –and not antagonism- of NMDA could be useful (Dhawan, Benveniste et al. 2011).

Cholinergic

On the basis of the role of the basal forebrain cholinergic system in motor learning and memory (Conner, Culberson et al. 2003), in saliency (Kleim and Jones 2008) and based on the experience with Alzheimer disease (Hansen, Gartlehner et al. 2008) different cholinesterase inhibitors have been tried with aphasic patients (Berthier, Pulvermuller et al. 2011).

In an open label study cholinergic agent donezepil was administered to 11 chronic post stoke aphasic patients: improved performances on the WAB-AQ was reported after 4 and 16 weeks but then declined with washout (Berthier, Hinojosa et al. 2003).

In another small open label study of 4 patients, the 2 patients receiving bifemelane increased their language scores (Tanaka, Miyazaki et al. 1997).

A double-blind, RCT combining donezepil versus placebo and SLT in 26 chronic aphasic patients, also showed a significant benefit of the donezepil group on language and communication measures (Berthier, Green et al. 2006).

Gabaergic

There is an anecdotic report of a chronic aphasic woman who improved transiently but, repetitively and dramatically her speech after zolpidem, an agonist of GABA receptor (Cohen, Chaaban et al. 2004).

In conclusion, despite evidence form basic science that certain drugs can promote plasticity, pharmacological intervention in aphasia has not conclusively proved its effectiveness; this is due mainly to poor study design, including patients with different types of aphasia and not using or describing homogeneous SLT associated with pharmacotherapy.

The time window of drug administration after stroke is probably important: in the acute phase preference would be given to drugs with neuroprotective effect or with potential to reestablish metabolic function whereas in the chronic phase preference would be given to drugs improving learning. Also, it seems that drugs should be given in association with SLT in view to obtain synergy between drug and behavioral therapies.

Transcranial Magnetic and Direct Current Stimulation

Another approach to SLT consists of favoring neuromodulation with transcranial brain stimulation. This kind of intervention has been carried out using non-invasive stimulation, such as transcranial magnetic or direct current stimulation. Although this kind of approach is still experimental at least regarding therapy for aphasia, a few studies have proposed transcranial stimulation with stroke patients either to suppress the potential inhibitory effect of the contra-lateral hemisphere or to enhance the excitability of perilesional areas. Here we will briefly review the outcome of studies using transcranial magnetic stimulation (TMS) or direct current stimulation (DCS) with aphasic participants.

Transcranial Magnetic Stimulation (TMS)

TMS is a non invasive technique consisting of a brief pulse of current flowing through a coil of wire and generating a magnetic field, which induces a physiological response in targeted brain regions. TMS applied repetitively (rTMS) can either inhibit or excite cortical activity depending on its frequency and intensity. Brain stimulation is used to increase cortical excitability aimed at facilitating long term potentiation like processes; inhibition is applied to the contralesional hemisphere in the aim to facilitate the ipsilesional hemisphere activity.

As excitatory high frequency TMS has safety issues in stroke patients (Tassinari, Cincotta et al. 2003), TMS has been applied mainly at low frequencies (1Hz) in order to disrupt locally cortical activity at right hemisphere areas potentially interfering with recovery in aphasic patients.

Preliminary experiments applied rTMS to suppress the unaffected right hemisphere in a small group of non-fluent aphasic patients (Martin, Naeser et al. 2004). These studies showed improvement in specific language production tasks, in particular when stimulation targeted the right Broca homologue area. The effects persisted two months after a 10 day treatment. The benefit in recovery has been assigned to a release of the affected left hemisphere from right hemispheric inhibition (Pascual-Leone, Amedi et al. 2005), (Bolognini, Pascual-Leone et al. 2009). Crucially, in the study by Naeser et al. improvement was observed only after stimulation of the right Broca homologue area, not after stimulation of right temporal areas. However, other studies have shown differential effects on a picture naming tasks when suppressing the right pars triangularis versus the right pars opercularis of the inferior frontal lobe (Naeser, Martin et al. 2011) or facilitative effects when excitatory stimulation was applied to these areas (Winhuisen, Thiel et al. 2005), suggesting a right hemispheric contribution to language recovery and questioning the general applicability of the inhibitory TMS approach (Turkeltaub, Coslett et al. 2011).

Direct Current Stimulation

Transcranial direct current stimulation (tDCS) is also a non-invasive brain polarisation technique that modulates the cortical excitability using weak direct currents. Depending on the polarity of the direct current (anodal vs.

cathodal) it increases or decreases brain excitability. Although its spatial and temporal resolution is lower than TMS, it is often preferred because it is safer and easier to use than TMS. In a few studies anodal tDCS applied to left perilesional areas showed positive effects on accuracy and latencies in picture naming tasks (Baker, Rorden et al. 2010), (Fridriksson, Richardson et al. 2011). Fridrikkson et al. (2011) applied anodal tDCS to left perilesional areas in association with computer-assisted therapy (CAT) sessions for anomia in eight chronic aphasic patients. They reported a decrease in production latencies relative to CAT sessions without tDCS. However, improvement has also been reported immediately after 10 minutes of tDCS without associated SLT (Monti, Cogiamanian et al. 2008). In this study cathodal tDCS applied to the left fronto-temporal areas in chronic non-fluent patients increased picture naming accuracy. The authors interpreted these results as an effect of decreased excitability of abnormal cortical inhibitory circuits. Alternatively, tDCS was applied to the right inferior frontal cortex (Vines, Norton et al. 2011). The authors investigated the effects of anodal tDCS in six chronic patients with non-fluent aphasia. tDCS stimulation was associated with three sessions of melodic intonation therapy. They reported greater improvement after the anodal tDCS relative to the therapy sessions without tDCS (sham).

In sum, both TMS and tDCS studies have shown some promising results in inducing long-lasting plastic changes and recovery in aphasic patients. So far, most studies have been conducted with chronic aphasic patients. At present however it is far from clear which brain areas should be targeted with excitatory vs. inhibitory stimulation. Actually, the type of SLT associated with cortical magnetic or electric stimulation or even inter-individual variability may modulate the choice of the targeted brain area, and this approach clearly needs additional empirical evidence before an extended application in clinical practice.

Conclusion

The basic knowledge of brain plasticity has grown but the exact mechanisms underlying recovery from aphasia are for the moment not fully understood and are a limit for the development of therapeutic option.

However today with certain evidence, a few recommendations can be retained.

The current practice of spreading SLT over a long period should be modified and short intensive treatment (massed practice) is preferred. There are a few methods which are indicated to increase treatment intensity: we have reviewed two of them: CIAT and CAT. These two treatment approaches have proved their efficacy and are certainly good candidates to address the issue of providing intensive treatment without increasing health costs. In all cases treated items in SLT should be chosen carefully because of the lack of generalization to untreated linguistic material and structures and the importance of having a relevant treatment.

Other approaches have emerged to facilitate neural plasticity and therefore improved treatment effects or recovery. Despite some encouraging results, these techniques still need to prove their efficacy. Importantly, if pharmacological or brain stimulation approaches are used, they should be coupled with adequate SLT, as they probably prime (re)learning, and learning cannot be achieved without training.

In sum, clinical practice has evolved during the past 20 years in several different directions to optimize SLT and its outcome; but most of these options still need to be better defined and developed.

References

Albert, M. L., D. L. Bachman, et al. (1988). "Pharmacotherapy for aphasia." *Neurology* 38(6): 877-879.

Ashtary, F., M. Janghorbani, et al. (2006). "A randomized, double-blind trial of bromocriptine efficacy in nonfluent aphasia after stroke." *Neurology* 66(6): 914-916.

Baker, J. M., C. Rorden, et al. (2010). "Using transcranial direct-current stimulation to treat stroke patients with aphasia." *Stroke* 41(6): 1229-1236.

Barrett, A. M. and P. J. Eslinger (2007). "Amantadine for adynamic speech: possible benefit for aphasia?" *Am J Phys Med Rehabil* 86(8): 605-612.

Berridge, K. C. and T. E. Robinson (1998). "What is the role of dopamine in reward: hedonic impact, reward learning, or incentive salience?" *Brain Res Brain Res Rev* 28(3): 309-369.

Berthier, M. L. (2005). "Poststroke Aphasia: Epidemiology, Pathophysiology and Treatment." *Drugs & Aging* 22(2): 163-182.

Berthier, M. L., C. Green, et al. (2006). "A randomized, placebo-controlled study of donepezil in poststroke aphasia." *Neurology* 67(9): 1687-1689.

Berthier, M. L., C. Green, et al. (2009). "Memantine and constraint-induced aphasia therapy in chronic poststroke aphasia." *Ann Neurol* 65(5): 577-585.

Berthier, M. L., J. Hinojosa, et al. (2003). "Open-label study of donezepil in chronic post stroke aphasia." *Neurology*: 128, 1219.

Berthier, M. L. and F. Pulvermuller (2011). "Neuroscience insights improve neurorehabilitation of poststroke aphasia." *Nat Rev Neurol* 7(2): 86-97.

Berthier, M. L., F. Pulvermuller, et al. (2011). "Drug therapy of post-stroke aphasia: a review of current evidence." *Neuropsychol Rev* 21(3): 302-317.

Bhogal, S. K., R. Teasell, et al. (2003). "Intensity of aphasia therapy, impact on recovery." *Stroke* 34(4): 987-993.

Bolognini, N., A. Pascual-Leone, et al. (2009). "Using non-invasive brain stimulation to augment motor training-induced plasticity." *J Neuroeng Rehabil* 6: 8.

Bragoni, M., M. Altieri, et al. (2000). "Bromocriptine and speech therapy in non-fluent chronic aphasia after stroke." *Neurol Sci* 21(1): 19-22.

Breitenstein, C., S. Wailke, et al. (2004). "D-amphetamine boosts language learning independent of its cardiovascular and motor arousing effects." *Neuropsychopharmacology* 29(9): 1704-1714.

Cherney, L., J. Patterson, et al. (2011). "Intensity of Aphasia Therapy: Evidence and Efficacy." *Current Neurology and Neuroscience Reports* 11(6): 560-569.

Cherney, L. R., J. P. Patterson, et al. (2008). "Evidence-Based Systematic Review: Effects of Intensity of Treatment and Constraint-Induced Language Therapy for Individuals With Stroke-Induced Aphasia." *J Speech Lang Hear Res* 51(5): 1282-1299.

Cicerone, K. D., C. Dahlberg, et al. (2005). "Evidence-based cognitive rehabilitation: updated review of the literature from 1998 through 2002." *Arch Phys Med Rehabil* 86(8): 1681-1692.

Cohen, L., B. Chaaban, et al. (2004). "Transient Improvement of Aphasia with Zolpidem." *New England Journal of Medicine* 350(9): 949-950.

Conner, J. M., A. A. Chiba, et al. (2005). "The Basal Forebrain Cholinergic System Is Essential for Cortical Plasticity and Functional Recovery following Brain Injury." *Neuron* 46(2): 173-179.

Conner, J. M., A. Culberson, et al. (2003). "Lesions of the Basal Forebrain Cholinergic System Impair Task Acquisition and Abolish Cortical Plasticity Associated with Motor Skill Learning." *Neuron* 38(5): 819-829.

Crerar, M. A., A. W. Ellis, et al. (1996). "Remediation of sentence processing deficits in aphasia using a computer-based microworld." *Brain Lang* 52(1): 229-275.

De Deyn, P. P., J. De Reuck, et al. (1997). "Treatment of Acute Ischemic Stroke With Piracetam." *Stroke* 28(12): 2347-2352.

Dhawan, J., H. Benveniste, et al. (2011). "A new look at glutamate and ischemia: NMDA agonist improves long-term functional outcome in a rat model of stroke." *Future Neurol* 6(6): 823-834.

Enderby, P., J. Broeckx, et al. (1994). "Effect of piracetam on recovery and rehabilitation after stroke: a double-blind, placebo-controlled study." *Clin Neuropharmacol* 17(4): 320-331.

Engelter, S. T., M. Gostynski, et al. (2006). "Epidemiology of aphasia attributable to first ischemic stroke: incidence, severity, fluency, etiology, and thrombolysis." *Stroke* 37(6): 1379-1384.

Faroqi-Shah, Y. and C. R. Virion (2009). "Constraint-induced language therapy for agrammatism: role of grammatical contraints." *Aphasiology* 23(7-8): 977-988.

Fink, R., A. Brecher, et al. (2002). "A computer-implemented protocol for treatment of naming disorders: evaluation of clinician-guided and partially self-guided instructions." *Aphasiology* 16: 1061-1086.

Floel, A., C. Breitenstein, et al. (2005). "Dopaminergic influences on formation of a motor memory." *Ann Neurol* 58(1): 121-130.

Fridriksson, J., J. D. Richardson, et al. (2011). "Transcranial direct current stimulation improves naming reaction time in fluent aphasia: a double-blind, sham-controlled study." *Stroke* 42(3): 819-821.

Gold, M., D. VanDam, et al. (2000). "An open-label trial of bromocriptine in nonfluent aphasia: a qualitative analysis of word storage and retrieval." *Brain Lang* 74(2): 141-156.

Gungor, L., M. Terzi, et al. (2011). "Does long term use of piracetam improve speech disturbances due to ischemic cerebrovascular diseases?" *Brain Lang* 117(1): 23-27.

Gupta, S. R., A. G. Mlcoch, et al. (1995). "Bromocriptine treatment of nonfluent aphasia." *Neurology* 45(12): 2170-2173.

Hansen, R. A., G. Gartlehner, et al. (2008). "Efficacy and safety of donepezil, galantamine, and rivastigmine for the treatment of Alzheimer's disease: a systematic review and meta-analysis." *Clin Interv Aging* 3(2): 211-225.

Hauk, O., I. Johnsrude, et al. (2004). "Somatotopic representation of action words in human motor and premotor cortex." *Neuron* 41(2): 301-307.

Huber, W. (1999). "The role of piracetam in the treatment of acute and chronic aphasia." *Pharmacopsychiatry* 32 Suppl 1: 38-43.

Huber, W., K. Willmes, et al. (1997). "Piracetam as an adjuvant to language therapy for aphasia: a randomized double-blind placebo-controlled pilot study." *Arch Phys Med Rehabil* 78(3): 245-250.

Jay, T. M. (2003). "Dopamine: a potential substrate for synaptic plasticity and memory mechanisms." *Prog Neurobiol* 69(6): 375-390.

Kelly, H., M. C. Brady, et al. (2010). "Speech and language therapy for aphasia following stroke." *Cochrane Database Syst Rev*(5): CD000425.

Kelly, H., M. C. Brady, et al. (2010). "Speech and language therapy for aphasia following stroke." *The Cochrane Library*(7).

Kessler, J., A. Thiel, et al. (2000). "Piracetam improves activated blood flow and facilitates rehabilitation of poststroke aphasic patients." *Stroke* 31(9): 2112-2116.

Kleim, J. A. and T. A. Jones (2008). "Principles of experience-dependent neural plasticity: implications for rehabilitation after brain damage." *J Speech Lang Hear Res* 51(1): S225-239.

Knecht, S., C. Breitenstein, et al. (2004). "Levodopa: faster and better word learning in normal humans." *Ann Neurol* 56(1): 20-26.

Laganaro, M., M. Di Pietro, et al. (2003). "Computerised treatment of anomia in chronic and acute aphasia: an exploratory study." *Aphasiology* 17: 709-721.

Laganaro, M., M. Di Pietro, et al. (2006a). "Computerised treatment of anomia in acute aphasia: treatment intensity and training size." *Neuropsychol Rehabil* 16(6): 630-640.

Laganaro, M., Di Pietro, M, et al.. (2006b). "What does recovery from anomia tell us about the underlying impairment: the case of similar anomic patterns and different recovery.". *Neuropsychologia* 44: 534-545.

Laganaro, M. and M. Overton Venet (2001). "Acquired alexia in multilingual aphasia and computer-assisted treatment in both languages: issues of generalisation and transfer." *Folia Phoniatr Logop* 53(3): 135-144.

Laska, A. C., M. von Arbin, et al. (2005). "Long-term antidepressant treatment with moclobemide for aphasia in acute stroke patients: a randomised, double-blind, placebo-controlled study." *Cerebrovasc Dis* 19(2): 125-132.

Leemann, B., M. Laganaro, et al. (2011). "Crossover trial of subacute computerized aphasia therapy for anomia with the addition of either levodopa or placebo." *Neurorehabil Neural Repair* 25(1): 43-47.

Maher, L. M., D. Kendall, et al. (2006). "A pilot study of use-dependent learning in the context of Constraint Induced Language Therapy." *J Int Neuropsychol Soc* 12(6): 843-852.

Malykh, A. G. and M. R. Sadaie (2010). "Piracetam and piracetam-like drugs: from basic science to novel clinical applications to CNS disorders." *Drugs* 70(3): 287-312.

Martin, P. I., M. A. Naeser, et al. (2004). "Transcranial magnetic stimulation as a complementary treatment for aphasia." *Semin Speech Lang* 25(2): 181-191.

Martinsson, L., H. Hardemark, et al. (2007). "Amphetamines for improving recovery after stroke." *Cochrane Database Syst Rev*(1): CD002090.

Meinzer, M., D. Djundja, et al. (2005). "Long-Term Stability of Improved Language Functions in Chronic Aphasia After Constraint-Induced Aphasia Therapy." *Stroke* 36(7): 1462-1466.

Meinzer, M., A. D. Rodriguez, et al. (2012). "First Decade of Research on Constrained-Induced Treatment Approaches for Aphasia Rehabilitation." *Arch Phys Med Rehabil* 93(1, Supplement): S35-S45.

Monti, A., F. Cogiamanian, et al. (2008). "Improved naming after transcranial direct current stimulation in aphasia." *J Neurol Neurosurg Psychiatry* 79(4): 451-453.

Mortley, J., P. Enderby, et al. (2001). "Using a computer to improve functional writing in a patient with severe dysgraphia." *Aphasiology* 15: 443-461.

Mortley, J., J. Wade, et al. (2004). "Superhighway to promoting a clinet-therapist partnership? Using the internet to deliver word-retrieval computer therapy, monitored remotely with minimal speech and language therapy input." *Aphasiology* 3: 193-211.

Naeser, M. A., P. I. Martin, et al. (2011). "TMS suppression of right pars triangularis, but not pars opercularis, improves naming in aphasia." *Brain Lang* 119(3): 206-213.

Noble, S. and P. Benfield (1998). "Piracetam. A review of its clinical potential in the managament of patients with stroke." *CNS Drugs*(6): 497-511.

Orgogozo, J. M. (1999). "Piracetam in the treatment of acute stroke." *Pharmacopsychiatry* 32 Suppl 1: 25-32.

Ozeren, A., Y. Sarica, et al. (1995). "Bromocriptine is ineffective in the treatment of chronic nonfluent aphasia." *Acta Neurol Belg* 95(4): 235-238.

Pascual-Leone, A., A. Amedi, et al. (2005). "The plastic human brain cortex." *Annu Rev Neurosci* 28: 377-401.

Pedersen, P., K. Vinter, et al. (2001). "Improvement of oral naming by unsupervised computerised rehabilitation." *Aphasiology* 15: 151-169.

Pulvermuller, F. and M. L. Berthier (2008). "Aphasia therapy on a neuroscience basis." *Aphasiology* 22(6): 563-599.

Pulvermuller, F., B. Neininger, et al. (2001). "Constraint-induced therapy of chronic aphasia after stroke." *Stroke* 32(7): 1621-1626.

Raymer, A. M., P. Beeson, et al. (2008). "Translational research in aphasia: from neuroscience to neurorehabilitation." *Journal of speech, language and hearing research* 51(S): 259-275.

Robertson, I. (1990). "Does computerized cognitive rehabilitation work? A review." *Aphasiology* 4: 381-405.

Rosser, N., P. Heuschmann, et al. (2008). "Levodopa improves procedural motor learning in chronic stroke patients." *Arch Phys Med Rehabil* 89(9): 1633-1641.

Sabe, L., R. Leiguarda, et al. (1992). "An open-label trial of bromocriptine in nonfluent aphasia." *Neurology* 42(8): 1637-1638.

Saur, D. and G. Hartwigsen (2012). "Neurobiology of language recovery after stroke: lessons from neuroimaging studies." *Arch Phys Med Rehabil* 93(1 Suppl): S15-25.

Scheidtmann, K., W. Fries, et al. (2001). "Effect of levodopa in combination with physiotherapy on functional motor recovery after stroke: a prospective, randomised, double-blind study." *Lancet* 358(9284): 787-790.

Seniow, J., M. Litwin, et al. (2009). "New approach to the rehabilitation of post-stroke focal cognitive syndrome: effect of levodopa combined with speech and language therapy on functional recovery from aphasia." *J Neurol Sci* 283(1-2): 214-218.

Sonde, L. and J. Lokk (2007). "Effects of amphetamine and/or L-dopa and physiotherapy after stroke - a blinded randomized study." *Acta Neurol Scand* 115(1): 55-59.

Stroemer, R. P., T. A. Kent, et al. (1998). "Enhanced neocortical neural sprouting, synaptogenesis, and behavioral recovery with D-amphetamine therapy after neocortical infarction in rats." *Stroke* 29(11): 2381-2393; discussion 2393-2385.

Tanaka, Y., M. Miyazaki, et al. (1997). "Effects of increased cholinergic activity on naming in aphasia." *Lancet* 350(9071): 116-117.

Tassinari, C. A., M. Cincotta, et al. (2003). "Transcranial magnetic stimulation and epilepsy." *Clin Neurophysiol* 114(5): 777-798.

Taub, E., G. Uswatte, et al. (1999). "Constraint-Induced Movement Therapy: a new family of techniques with broad application to physical rehabilitation--a clinical review." *J Rehabil Res Dev* 36(3): 237-251.

Thompson, C. K. (2000). "The neurobiology of language recovery in aphasia." *Brain Lang* 71(1): 245-248.

Turkeltaub, P. E., H. B. Coslett, et al. (2011). "The right hemisphere is not unitary in its role in aphasia recovery." *Cortex*.

Vines, B. W., A. C. Norton, et al. (2011). "Non-invasive brain stimulation enhances the effects of melodic intonation therapy." *Front Psychol* 2: 230.

Walker-Batson, D., S. Curtis, et al. (2001). "A double-blind, placebo-controlled study of the use of amphetamine in the treatment of aphasia." *Stroke* 32(9): 2093-2098.

Wertz, R. and R. Katz (2004). "Outcome of computer treatment for aphasia." *Aphasiology* 18: 229-244.

Whiting, E., H. J. Chenery, et al. (2007). "Dexamphetamine boosts naming treatment effects in chronic aphasia." *Journal of the international neuropsychological society.* 13: 972-979.

Whiting, E., H. J. Chenery, et al. (2008). "The explicit learning of new names for known objects is improved by dexamphetamine." *Brain Lang* 104(3): 254-261.

Winhuisen, L., A. Thiel, et al. (2005). "Role of the contralateral inferior frontal gyrus in recovery of language function in poststroke aphasia: a combined repetitive transcranial magnetic stimulation and positron emission tomography study." *Stroke* 36(8): 1759-1763.

In: Aphasia   ISBN: 978-1-62257-681-4
Editors: E. Holmgren, E.S. Rudkilde   © 2013 Nova Science Publishers, Inc.

Chapter IV

Diagnosis and Management of Language Impairment in Acute Stroke

Constance Flamand-Roze[1,*], Heather Flowers[2], Emmanuel Roze[3] and Christian Denier[1,4,5]
[1]Department of Neurology, Centre Hospitalo-Universitaire
de Bicêtre, Assistance Publique – Hôpitaux de Paris,
Le Kremlin Bicêtre, France
[2]Department of Speech Language Pathology,
University of Toronto, Canada
[3]Department of Neurology, Salpêtrière Hospital,
Assistance Publique - Hôpitaux de Paris, Paris, France
[4]PARIS Sud XI University, France
[5]INSERM 4788, Le Kremlin Bicêtre, France

Abstract

Language impairments are frequent in stroke, especially in the hyper acute phase, occurring in 15 to 50% of stroke patients. Recovery from aphasia remains difficult to predict. Language impairment still exists in at

*   E-mails: constance.flamand-roze@bct.aphp.fr., heather.flowers@utoronto.ca, emmanuel.
    flamand-roze@psl.aphp.fr., christian.denier@bct.aphp.fr. Tel: +33 1 45 21 26 18. Fax: + 33
    1 45 21 28 53.

least 50% of initially aphasic patients one year after stroke. Post-stroke aphasia is a major source of disability that can lead to impaired communication, reduced social activities, depression and a decreased likelihood of resuming work. The role of the stroke unit in improving morbidity, mortality and recovery has been clearly demonstrated. Nevertheless, the need for intense and sustained acute management of aphasia in specialized stroke units remains controversial. The recent validation of a tool to rapidly screen for aphasia (LAST) after stroke allows for its early detection and management. Early detection of aphasia after stroke may improve outcomes by taking advantage of the synergy between intensive speech therapy and early neural reorganization. Daily re-evaluation will facilitate tailored rehabilitation sessions, multidisciplinary management by the stroke team, and development of educational resources for patients and their caregivers. Standardizing protocols for identifying and managing aphasia requires the co-operation and coordination of the entire stroke team, along with the daily presence of speech therapists. These considerations are crucial for patients in the stroke unit to achieve the full benefit of the management proposed in this chapter, to ultimately promote better long term functional prognosis.

Introduction

Stroke is a public health issue, representing the third leading cause of death and the first leading cause of disability in adults [1] in the western world. As the population ages, its estimated incidence of 300 to 500/100 000 is expected to increase [2]. Specialized stroke units and/or stroke teams have been created worldwide in order to provide optimized management of stroke in the hyper acute and acute stages. Recent randomized controlled trials (RCT) have proven the efficiency of specialized stroke units in reducing morbidity and mortality, and in facilitating rapid recuperation after stroke [3-6]. Aphasia is a frequent symptom of acute stroke, and a major source of disability. It incurs increased cost of care [7] and has negative economic repercussions, such as decreased return to work [8,9]. However, early intense and sustained management of aphasia in stroke units remains controversial.

We share herein our experience of the early identification and treatment of aphasia after stroke, based primarily on a neurolinguistic framework. We further describe existing protocols and discuss the expected benefits of early management. Optimal standardization of aphasia management can be achieved in stroke units with collaboration among physicians, nurses and speech therapists, resulting in improved outcomes after stroke.

Moreover, clinically-driven research in aphasia in the acute setting is feasible and essential to improving recovery and rehabilitation outcomes.

1. Impairments in the Acute Phase of Stroke: Generalities

Survivors of stroke often experience multiple co-occurring impairments, such as hemiplegia [10,11] dysphagia [12, 13], incontinence [14,15] depression [16], cognitive changes [17,18], dysarthria [19,20] and/or language impairment [21,22]. Second to hemiparesis, dysphagia, dysarthria, and language impairment are the most frequent [20]. The incidence of dysphagia approximates 55% in the acute stage [12,13]. Dysarthria and language impairment are almost as frequent in the acute phase of stroke, occurring in approximatively one-third of all stroke patients. Nonetheless, these impairments are probably underestimated, particularly in the hyper acute stage, given the lack of standardized assessments and the potential for rapid recovery [21, 23-25]. Dysarthria may occur as isolated speech impairment or with concomitant aphasia. Studies have reported dysarthria to range from 8 [26] to 42% [19] and aphasia to range from15 [24] to 41% [12] following stroke. Inclusion of different stroke etiologies, first versus recurrent stroke patients and different methodologies likely contributes to variations in reported frequencies of language impairment.

1.1. Definitions

Stroke is usually defined as a sudden onset of signs of focal disturbance of cerebral function lasting over 24 hours [27]. Language impairment literature can relate to ischemic, intracerebral hemorrhage (ICH) or subarachnoid hemorrhage (SAH) stroke etiologies.

Among stroke subtypes, ischemic etiology is the most frequent cause of stroke, followed by ICH and then SAH [28-30]. While there is typically an abrupt onset of neurological deficit after ischemic stroke, a progressive evolution, often with considerable tissue displacement [31], can also exist after ICH [26].

In addition, there is as much as a 10 fold higher frequency of decreased level of consciousness after ICH compared to ischemic stroke [26]. Consequently, aphasia can be identified very early after ischemic stroke, while patients with ICH may require ongoing monitoring for adequate identification of its presence. After ischemic stroke, some patients may fully recover from aphasia within days of stroke onset [24], thereby warranting careful monitoring for early recovery. Aphasia and other focal neurological deficits are not generally expected to occur after SAH, except occasionally as transient signs of vasospasm [30], or after aneurysm clipping [32]. Aphasia or language impairment is defined as an acquired impairment, characterized by anomia [33] and/or other deficits in expressive or receptive language, evidenced in any modality: speaking, listening, reading, or writing [34]. We use a neurolinguistic framework to describe brain behavior relationships in the identification and management of language impairment after stroke.(figure 1)

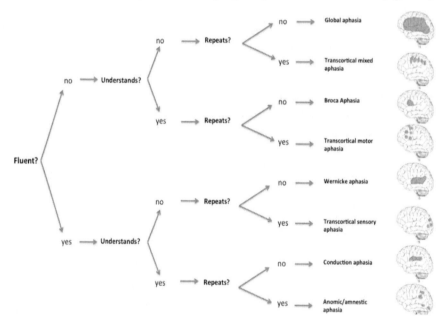

Figure 1. Decision-making tree in aphasic patients.

1.2. Incidence, Predictors and Phenotypes of Language Impairment

Aphasia results from injury to the dominant hemisphere, which involves the left hemisphere in right-handed patients and in 70% of left-handed patients [35,36]. The neural network subserving language function is increasingly recognized to be a large and complex system involving regions throughout the cerebral hemisphere. The language network comprises areas of the perisylvian cortex, including the classical language areas of Broca and Wernicke: Broca's area or Brodmann's area 44 in the posterior inferior frontal gyrus innervates adjacent motor neurons subserving the mouth and larynx, and controls the output of spoken language; Wernicke's area or Brodmann's area 22, comprising the posterior two-thirds of the superior temporal gyrus, receives information from the auditory cortex and accesses a network of cortical associations to assign word meanings; the angular gyrus in the inferior parietal lobule is adjacent to visual receptive areas and subserves the perception of written language, as well as other language processing functions. Additional regions have a significant contribution to language function: the insula, several frontal and temporal lobe regions and vast regions of the temporal, occipital, and parietal cortex, as well as subcortical nuclei. [37-42]

The incidence of aphasia may differ according to stroke etiology (see table 1). Some studies have documented aphasia in unselected stroke samples, involving all three etiologies: ischemic, ICH and SAH, with frequencies ranging between 21%[43] and 35% [44]. Samples that considered only first-ever stroke for all three etiologies have reported frequencies ranging from 17 [45] to 30% [46]. When SAH was excluded, studies have reported frequencies ranging from 23 [43] to 41% [12]. To our knowledge, only two studies have included both types of hemorrhagic stroke, reporting a combined frequency of 9% [43] and 20% [47]. After isolated ICH, the reported frequency of aphasia ranges from 15 [48] to 36% [12]. Two studies have reported aphasia frequencies of 3 [12] and 12% [31] after SAH. Documents of the frequency of aphasia after ischemic stroke range from 15 [24] to 40% [12], with frequencies ranging from 23 [20] to 39% [37] after first ischemic stroke. The presence of language impairment is preferentially associated with previous stroke [12], increasing age [12,21,22,41,42] female gender [42], stroke severity [24], atrial fibrillation [21,22,49,50], cardio-embolic etiology [51]. Published reports differ concerning the frequency of phenotypes of aphasia after stroke and there is a paucity of literature describing the clinico-radiological correlation. Croquelois and Bogousslavsky recently studied 1541 patients with aphasia in the early stages of stroke (ie within the 24 hours following onset), classifying them according to aphasic patterns, where 38% presented with expressive-receptive aphasia, 37% with expressive aphasia and 25% with receptive aphasia [52] (see figure 2). In same setting, Kumral and his colleagues described a series of 454 patients with acute aphasia in the first four weeks after stroke, identifying receptive-expressive aphasia in 60%, expressive aphasia in 22%, and receptive aphasia in 14% [30].

Table 1. Frequency of Acute Aphasia according Stroke Etiology, by increasing frequency

Study	Frequency %	Sample n	Assessing Health Professional
MIXED ETIOLOGIES			
All Etiologies			
Hilari* (2011)	17	12	unclear
Hier et al[a] (1994)	21	1805	neurologist
Inzitari et al (1998)	22	339	physician
Kumral et al*[b] (1988)	23	2000	neurologist
Kyrozis et al* (2009)	23	555	physician
Lawrence et al* (2001)	23	1259	physician
Bersano et al (2009)	28	8848	neurologist
Stegmayr et al* (1994)	30	3542	medical staff
Sturmer et al[b] (2002)	31	270	physician
Dickey et al[c] (2010)	35	3207	stroke care team or CNS
ISCH and ICH			
Hier et al (1994)	23	1510	neurologist
Croquelois & Bogousslavsky* (2011)	26	5880	physician
Hilari* (2011)	33	96	unclear
Laska et al (2001)	33	106	SLT
Bogousslavsky et al* (1998)	34	1000	unclear
Guyomard et al[d] (2009)	41	2983	physician or nurse
ICH and SAH			
Hier et al[a] (1994)	9	490	neurologist
Sturmer et al (2002)	20	50	physician
ISOLATED ETIOLOGIES			
ICH			
Bahou[e] (2009)	15	100	physician
Hier et al (1994)	16	237	neurologist
Croquelois & Bogousslavsky* (2011)	26	647	physician
Bersano et al (2009)	32	1009	neurologist
Guyomard et al (2009)	36	314	physician or nurse
SAH			
Hier et al[a] (1994)	3	243	neurologist
Anderson et al[f] (2006)	12	868	neuropsychologist
ISCH			
Inatomi et al[g] (2008)	15	835	neurologist or SLT
Lubart et al*[h] (2005)	23	140	neurologist
Hier et al (1994)	24	1273	neurologist
Croquelois & Bogousslavsky* (2011)	26	5233	physician
Engelter et al* (2006)	30	269	neurologist
Sturmer et al[b] (2002)	34	220	physician
Hilari* (2011)	39	76	unclear
Guyomard et al (2009)	40	2318	physician or nurse

Abreviations: CNS= Canadian Neurological Scale.; ICH=Intracerebral Haemorrhage; ISCH=Ischemic Etiology; SAH=Subarachnoid Haemorrhage; SLT=Speech Language Therapist; * first ever stroke.; (a)proportion of SAH higher than that of ICH.; (b)TIA included in ischemic category.(c)35% incidence documented at discharge, compared to 30% very early after stroke;(d)included ISCH, ICH, and undetermined etiology; (e)Excluded cerebral trauma as cause of ICH;(f)Used a cueed word finding task; combined results for those with hypothermia and those with normothermia; (g)Only included patients with good premorbid activities of daily living; (h)Geriatric ward sample of older patients.

Two studies have described more specific phenotypes in series of consecutively admitted patients with aphasia [23, 25] (see figure 2), where one demonstrated the highest frequency for expressive-receptive aphasia [23] and the other for expressive aphasia [25]. In both studies, receptive aphasia types were least frequent [23,25]. Two additional studies have reported subtypes of aphasia in acute stroke patients following ischemic stroke and ICH, excluding SAH [43, 53]. In one of these two studies, expressive-receptive aphasia predominated [43] at 40%, while receptive aphasia was most frequent in the other [53] at 65%. The small sample size in the latter study may account for this variation [53], when compared to the larger studies.

Three studies have considered aphasia classifications after isolated etiologies. Two documented aphasia after ischemic etiology [24,43], demonstrating that expressive-receptive aphasia predominated, with frequencies of 41% [43] and 56% [24], followed by expressive aphasia with frequencies of 27% [43] and 29% [24]. Receptive aphasia was least frequent at 14% in both studies.

Hier and his colleagues also documented aphasia subtypes after intracerebral hemorrhage, demonstrating the highest frequency for receptive-expressive aphasia at 31%, followed by expressive aphasia at 27% and then receptive aphasia at 14% [43].

Discrepancies in these results are probably due to differences between the sensitivity and specificity of tools versus bedside clinical evaluation and to the timing of evaluation, as aphasia can improve rapidly shortly after the onset of stroke.

To illustrate, a study involving 130 acute ischemic stroke patients with aphasia demonstrated improvement of aphasia in 46% and resolution in 21% within the first 10 days following stroke onset [24]. In addition to reporting aphasia based on subtypes in these studies, some authors noted numerous unclassifiable aphasias (25%) [23, 43] or subcortical aphasias [23]. These unclassifiable aphasias may be comprised of patients with co-occurring subtypes or they may result from the method of determining subtypes, where certain patients do not fit the study's definition of each subtype.

Also, diaschisis and "penumbra phenomenon", resulting in hypoperfusion to anatomical regions associated with aphasia, are possible explanations for rapid improvement, subcortical aphasia [23] or for evolution from nonfluent to fluent aphasia [25].

Mixed Etiologies

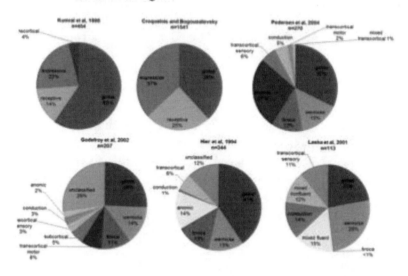

Isolated Etiologies – Ischemic Stroke

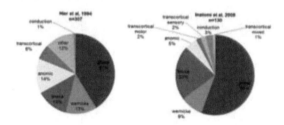

Isolated Etiologies –Intracerebral Hemorrhage

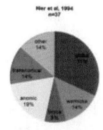

Figure 2. Classification of aphasia subtypes according to stroke etiologies by study. Total percentages may not equal one hundred, due to rounding to the nearest percent.

1.3. Prognosis

In spite of the potential for rapid improvement, language impairment usually still affects 50% of initially aphasic patients 18 months after stroke [25,53], thereby contributing to altered quality of life beyond the aphasia itself [45]. Primary consequences may include symptoms of depression, difficulty to participating in rehabilitation, difficulty understanding therapists', social draw-back and decreased frequency of professional activities [54-56].

It is difficult to predict the outcome of aphasia, even if aphasia after hemorrhagic stroke has a better prognosis than after cerebral infarctions [57]. To the present day, only initial stroke severity (according to NIHSS) and the initial severity of aphasia have been shown to predict importance of aphasia recovery after acute ischemic stroke [24,25]. In a recent study, Maas conclude that advanced age, the presence of hypodense regions, a history of previous stroke, and sedentary activity level significantly predicted a diminished likelihood of language improvement at discharge. At 6 months of follow-up, only the prestroke mRS significantly impacted likelihood of improvement [58].

2. Tools for Language Assessment

2.1. Available Tools

Early detection of aphasia after stroke may improve rehabilitation by taking advantage of the synergy between intensive speech therapy and early neural reorganization [59-61]. Tools capable of detecting aphasia and evaluating its severity during the acute phase of stroke might help to improve early rehabilitation and to predict outcome [62]. Standard aphasia rating scales such as the Western Aphasia Battery, the Boston Diagnostic Aphasia Evaluation (BDAE), and the Boston Naming Test are not appropriate for use during the acute phase of stroke [61,63-65]. In particular, these gold standard test batteries take too long to complete and must be administered by speech and language therapists [63-65]. Global stroke rating scales such as the National Institutes of Health Stroke Scale and the Scandinavian Stroke Scale include language items and have been developed for use in acute settings [66-71], but they do not reliably detect aphasia [62]. Several attempts have been made to develop and validate brief aphasia screening scales suitable for patients with acute stroke [72-79], but all have inherent structural limitations, including [61]: (1) inclusion of written language subtests, the results of which are influenced by hemiplegia and illiteracy [59,73-76,79]; (2) use of complex visual material inappropriate for stroke patients with neuro-visual deficits [73,74], (3) inclusion of subtests that are markedly influenced by attention/executive dysfunction [73,74]; (4) excessively lengthy administration [76] ; (5) difficulties with administration or scoring [59,72,76,79]; and (6) IQ dependency [75]. Some of these scales also have poor sensitivity for the detection of aphasia and a provide little information regarding measures of validity and reliability [59,76].

2.2. A Novel Tool: LAST, the Language Screening Test

Early and precise diagnosis of aphasia is necessary and justified for informed decision making, such as the use of thrombolysis and the implementation of early and individually-tailored rehabilitation. Evaluation may help to localize lesion site, prior to magnetic resonance imaging [80]. A quantitative tool is needed to document the risk or presence of aphasia and toquantify repeat evaluations. Such a tool would also permit description of aphasic patterns according to lesion localization, such as transcortical aphasia following acute border-zone infarcts [81,82]. A recent study investigated the correlation between language tasks and brain lesions, concluding that word repetition, sentence repetition and naming best-predicted lesions in the left hemisphere lesion [83]. Counting and comprehension were also impaired in patients with brain injuries [83].

We recently developed and validated a brief language screening scale in French, the Language Screening Test (LAST) [84], to screen for risk of aphasia and to facilitate timely assessment of patients after acute stroke. We validated and documented reliability for two versions of the tool in an unselected sample of chronic and acute stroke patients, excluding SAH. The scale consists of 5 subtests: picture naming (items selected based on lexical familiarity and image evoking value), repetition (of a word and a sentence), automatic sequence (counting from 1 to 10), picture recognition (including semantic, visual and phonemic foils) and auditory commands (including 1 simple and 2 complex instructions). These subtests were chosen for their high correlation with left hemisphere lesions. Two parallel and equivalent versions of LAST (a and b) were developed to avoid a re-test effect. Each items is scored as 1 if correct and 0 if incorrect or inappropriate; The total scores ranges from 0 to 15, with a cut-off at 14 for the diagnosis of aphasia, as compared to the BDAE. The test is administered on a letter-sized sheet of paper (one side for the expressive index and one side for the receptive index). Administration requires fewer than three minutes. The simplicity of LAST makes it suitable for bedside administration by any health professional. The LAST is useful as a rapid and reliable screen for aphasia, with proven specificity. Given the existence of two parallel versions, a second quantification of aphasia is possible during a follow-up period.

3. Recovery

Speech and language therapy is assumed to be beneficial; A recent Cochrane review (2010) reported some indications of the effectiveness of SLT for people with aphasia following stroke[85]. Moreover, the authors documented results favouring intensive SLT over conventional SLT. However, there was insufficient evidence in this review to establish the effectiveness of one SLT approach over another [85].

Neural processes underlying recovery remain unknown [86]. Different factors may play a role, such as age, stroke size and location, premorbid level of education, and environmental support [63]. It has been documented that hemorrhagic strokes evolve better than ischemic strokes [57]. However, the only predictive factor of speech and language recovery following cerebral infarctions is the initial severity of stroke [24,25]. One study postulated that, as with motor recovery, improvement from aphasia is directly correlated with the initial deficiency, with an estimated recovery of 70% at 90 days post stroke onset [87].

Aphasia usually results from lesions affecting the left hemisphere in right-handed patients as well as in the majority of left-handed patients [35,36]. Cerebral plasticity and changes in neural organization interfere with the restoration of language function [88,89]. This is due to post-stroke compensation in the undamaged language areas, perilesional tissue and homologue right language areas [90]. In the setting of a very focal lesion, perilesional areas participate in recovery at the acute phase and during rehabilitation.

Two different mechanisms are supposed: transient hypoperfusion of these territories ("penumbra") and early neuronal reorganization with up regulation of these areas [91]. In larger lesions, language recovery could implicate the right hemisphere, as demonstrated in functional imaging and neurophysiologic studies [92-94]. Homologous right-sided regions that could be implicated in the process of language recovery are the superior temporal lobe (auditory control), the inferior frontal gyrus, pre-motor areas (planning of motor actions and nonlinguistic perception of language) and the motor cortex (execution of verbal motor actions) [86,95,96]. A recent study reports the extraordinary case of a man who benefited from a pre and post stroke functional MRI (fMRI): the patient presented with a Broca's aphasia after a large ischemic infarction within the territory of the left middle cerebral artery, with almost complete recovery [96].

The fMRI shows a perilesional reorganization but no significant recruitment of the right hemisphere one year after stroke [96]. A second functional MRI study reported the dynamics of language reorganization in 14 stroke patients describing activation of perilesional areas initially (as explored at day 2) [90]. Subsequent areas of reorganization included the right homologue of Broca's area in the sub acute period (day 12 after stroke) and later the reactivation of the left language areas in the chronic phase (explored one year after onset of symptoms) [90]. These findings should be taken in account when planning rehabilitation.

4. Rehabilitation

Speech and language therapy (SLT) aims at improving communication using verbal or nonverbal treatment modalities. Recent guidelines recommend speech therapy for patients with aphasia following stroke in spite of contradictory results from a few previous studies [85,97,98]. This heterogeneity could result from unsuitable tools, large heterogeneous cohorts, initiation of intensive therapy at differing time periods following stroke [99] or different rehabilitation techniques [98,100].

Functional imaging and behavioral studies have shown that SLT can modulate neural plasticity [101]. Because inappropriate rehabilitation may interfere with reorganization of language, it should be implemented according to the aphasia classification. Therefore, semantic phonological, and/or morphosyntactic therapies should be proposed according to the initial language impairment [102, 103]. In our center, different methods of SLT are performed according to each patient's needs and type of aphasia. We suggest that therapy should be implemented on a daily basis as early after stroke onset as possible. In particular, the specific contributions of the right hemisphere, such as prosodic and rhythmic properties of language, should be targeted in therapy to favor activation of controlateral language areas [104]. Early SLT in nonverbal patients or patients with severely reduced verbal output is important in order to avoid stereotypies. In accordance with one hypothesis on the dynamics of language recovery, and to capitalize on the potential role of the right hemisphere, we practice early SLT using melodic intonation therapy (MIT) [92]. We have proposed an auditory stimulation program, using a daily music listening program in our unit (one hour of music with French lyrics for our francophone population), derived from recently reported benefits [104]. Patients are encouraged to listen to music with lyrics and to actively sing along. A recent study with clinician blinding has sought to determine the immediate effects of introducing MIT early after stroke onset in patients with Broca's aphasia [105]. The treatment group showed a significant improvement compared to the control group, supporting the benefit of using this therapy method after acute stroke [105].

Although some have argued that early speech therapy is not feasible or necessary, we contend that it is indeed feasible and paramount to optimizing recovery. Second to promoting language recovery, initiation of therapy may reassure patients and help educate caregivers. As part of the therapeutic initiative, caregivers are provided advice for supportive communication [106] and to aid in eliciting compensatory strategies from the patient. Early therapy also facilitates better communication in patient care regarding medical explanations, instructions, and interactions with other therapists and the medical team.

Contribution from the entire medical and paramedical team is essential in the treatment of aphasia. In our stroke unit, therapeutic information is discussed with nursing staff, because their frequent patient interactions are crucial for progression toward rehabilitation goals. Their numerous daily interventions with patients may play a role in increasing the intensity and functionality of speech and language objectives. Providing adequate information about aphasia to front-line health professionals and families is essential to avoid ambiguous interactions. This will promote clear explanations conducive to the reception capabilities of patients. Similar educational information and explanations are necessary for both families and caregivers to avoid misconceptions. For example, some relatives may think that a patient has incurred hearing loss, amnesia, cognitive decline or dementia, psychiatric disorders or that the patient lacks physical sensation or emotion. Unfortunately, aphasia is not well understood, and educating family members and caregivers is essential to facilitate faster and more efficient recovery on the part of patients. Families and caregivers need to be well informed about the diagnosis and potential prognosis of the aphasia. As with front-line health care workers, other health professionals, such as physiotherapists or occupational therapists are inherently implicated in language rehabilitation in the acute phase. Their actions should be verbalized in an accessible formulation, with clear articulation, and with sufficient confirmation that the patient understands the instructions. In patients who are nonverbal or who have extremely limited verbal output, compensatory strategies such as the use of pictures, gestural communication, and letter require explanation to families and caregivers to prevent communication breakdown. Associated impairments, such as anosognosia after posteriorly localized aphasia and depression after anteriorly localized aphasia require additional considerations and caregiver education from the stroke team.

5. Perspectives

Effectiveness of SLT has been shown in different studies, and tools are now available to assess aphasia in acute stroke. Randomized controlled trials are still needed to indicate the best approach to delivering speech and language therapy. This will inform indications for the optimal approach, frequency, and duration of allocation and format of SLT for specific patient groups. Fortunately, recent randomized controlled studies have been conducted in the acute stage with a particular consideration of methods of speech therapy [103,107]. Controversy from potentially contradictory results arose from methodological differences such as group size, randomization methods, and type, timing (early vs. delayed) and frequency of therapy (intensive vs. conventional) [85, 98,108]. Intensive SLT, of any type, has been shown to be beneficial according to some authors [103]. Others consider that "intensive" and "early" SLT should be undertaken to promote early neuronal re-organization [59-61,103].

Considering different therapy types by SLTs, a recent RCT investigated the effect of "Language enrichment therapy" [107], starting at day 2 post stroke and continuing to day 21. The control group received no SLT for at least the first 21 days post stroke. At day 21, 58% of the treatment group achieved a higher score on the aphasia test battery, while 35% achieved higher scores in the control group. However, the treatment group did not maintain gains in verbal communication six months following stroke. A more recent pilot RCT evaluated daily SLT according to patient classifications of aphasia, involving linguistically driven therapeutic tasks [103]. They compared patient tailored therapy with usual care and found that patients in the treatment group had significantly higher scores on the aphasia quotient and on a functional communication measure than the usual care group. Additional RCTs are still needed to better determine the optimal type, timing and intensity of speech language therapy in the setting of acute stroke.

The validation and availability of the LAST and the recent demonstration of the feasibility of conducting RCTs in the very early stages of stroke provide the impetus for designing future randomized studies that take type, timing and intensity of SLT into account after acute stroke. In addition, use of a validated language scale, such as the LAST, in randomized trials or consecutive cohorts, could further promote research correlating acute clinical signs of aphasia with MRI, by which the efficacy of therapy for aphasia subtypes could be documented.

Conclusion

The early detection of aphasia after stroke is essential for reliable diagnosis in order to optimize rehabilitation. Available recent tools now allow for rapid and precise assessment of aphasia. Standard care protocols and teamwork promote best practice in the use of these tools, rendering them more efficient and effective. The implementation of such protocols involves the cooperation and coordination of both medical and paramedical personnel and the daily presence of speech therapists in stroke units. In particular, we recommend this daily presence for patients with aphasia, so that they may derive maximum benefit and the advantages of units that provide this type of standard care. Consequently, we expect that the long-term functional prognosis of these patients with aphasia will improve. Moreover, future randomized trials are essential to develop specific interventions for and to optimize SLT support.

References

[1]   Murray CJ, Lopez AD: Global mortality, disability, and the contribution of risk factors: Global Burden of Disease Study. *Lancet* 1997; 349:1436-1442.

[2]   Sudlow C.L.M., MRCP(UK); C.P. Warlow, FRCP; for the International Stroke Incidence Collaboration: Comparable Studies of the Incidence of

Stroke and its Pathological Types Results From an International Collaboration *Stroke* 1997;28:491-499.

[3] Indredavik B., Bakke F, Solberg R, et al.: Benefit of a stroke unit: a randomized controlled trial. *Stroke* 1991;22(8):1026-31.

[4] Indredavik B, Bakke F, SA, et al.: Stroke unit treatment improves long-term quality of life: a randomized controlled trial. *Stroke* 1998;29(5):895-9.

[5] Kalra L: The influence of stroke unit rehabilitation on functional recovery from stroke. *Stroke* 1994;25(4):821-5.

[6] Saposnik, G., Hassan, K. A., Selchen, D., Fang, J., Kapral, M. K., and Smith, E. E.: Stroke unit care: Does ischemic stroke subtype matter? *International Journal of Stroke* 2011;6(3), 244-250.

[7] Hellis C, Simpson AN, Bonilha H, Mauldin P.D, Simpson K.N: The one-year attributable cost of post stroke aphasia. *Stroke* 2012;43(5):1429-31.

[8] Ross-Graham J, Pereira S, Teasell R. Aphasia and return to work in younger stroke survivors. *Aphasiology* 2011;25(8) 952-960.

[9] Dalemans R.J.P, De Witte L.P, Wade D.T, Van den Heuvel W.A.A description of social participation in working-age persons with aphasia: a review of the literature. *Aphasiology* 2008;22(10):1071-1091.

[10] Mazaux J.M, Barat M, Borde Ch, Arne L. Disturbznces of the body schema during rehabilitation in hemiplegia. *Annales de Médecine Physique* 1980; 23(2): 248-255.

[11] Petrilli S, Durufle A, Nicolas B, Pinel J.F, Kerdoncuff V, Gallien P. Hemiplegia and return to domicile. *Annales de Médecine Physique et de Réadaptation* 2002;45(2):69-76.

[12] Guyomard V, Fulcher R.A, Redmayne O, Metcalf A.K, Potter J.F, Myint P.K. Effect of dysphasia and dysphagia on inpatient mortality and hospital lenght of stay: a database study. *Journal of the American Geriatric Society* 2009;57(11):2101-2106.

[13] Martino R, Foley N, Bhogal S, Diamant N, Speechley M, Teasell R. Dysphagia after stroke: incidence, diagnosis, and pulmonary complications. *Stroke* 2005; 36(12):2756-2763.

[14] Du G, Fu Q, Liu W. Prediction of urinary incontinence after cerebral infarction. 2005. *Chinese Journal of Clinical Rehabilitation* 2010; 9(29):10-11.

[15] Dumoulin C, Korner-Bitensky N, Tannenbaum C. Unrinary incontinence after stroke: identification, assessment and intervention by rehabilitation professionals in Canada. *Stroke* 2007; 38(10): 2745-2751.

[16] Carota A, Staub F, Bogousslavsky J. Emotions, behaviours and mood changes in stroke. *Current Opinion in Neurology* 2002; 15(1):57-69.

[17] Khateb A, Annoni J, Lopez U, Bernasconi F, Lavanchy L, Bogousslavsky J. Evaluation of cognitive and behavioural disorders in stroke unit. In O Godeffroy and J Bogousslavsky (Eds). 2007. The behavioural and cognitive neurology of stroke. 1-14. New York, NY, US: Cambridge University Press.

[18] Lesniak M, Bak T, Czepiel W, Seniow J, Czlonkowska A. Frequency and prognostic value of cognitive disorders in stroke patients. *Dementia and Geriatric Cognitive Disorders* 2008; 26(4): 356-363.

[19] Lawrence E.S, Coshall C, Dundas R, Stewart J, Rudd A.G, Howard R et al. Estimate of the prevalence of acute stroke impairments and disability in a multiethnic population. *Stroke*2001 ; 32(6): 1279-1284.

[20] Lubart E, Leibovitz A, Baumoehl Y, Klein C, Gil I, Abramovitz I et al. Progressing stroke with neurological deterioration in a group of israeli elderly. *Archives of Gerontology and Geriatrics* 2005 ; 41(1): 95-100.

[21] Engelter ST, Gostynski M, Papa S, et al.: Epidemiology of aphasia attributable to first ischemic stroke: incidence, severity, fluency, etiology, and thrombolysis. *Stroke* 2006;37(6):1379-84.

[22] Hillis ALE, Heilder J. Mechanisms of early aphasia recovery. *Aphasiology* 2002; 16(9): 885-895.

[23] Godefroy O, Dubois C, Debachy B, et al.: Vascular aphasias: main characteristics of patients hospitalized in acute stroke units. *Stroke* 2002;33(3):702-5.

[24] Inatomi Y, Yonehara T, Omiya S, et al.: Aphasia during the acute phase in ischemic stroke. *Cerebrovasc. Dis.* 2008;25(4):316-23.

[25] Pedersen PM, Vinter K, Olsen TS: Aphasia after stroke: type, severity and prognosis. The Copenhagen aphasia study. *Cerebrovasc. Dis.* 2004;17(1):35-43.

[26] Bogousslavsky J, Van Melle G, Regli F. The Lausanne stroke registery: analysis of 1000 consecutive patients with first stroke. *Stroke* 1988; 19(9): 1083-1092.

[27] Goldstein M, Barnett H.J.M, Orgogozo J.M, Sartorius N, Symon L, Vereschagin N.V. Report of the WHO task force on stroke and other cerebrovascular disorders. *International Journal of Language and Communication Disorders* 1989; 33 (supp): 158-161.

[28] Broderick JP, Brott T, Tomsick T, Miller R, Huster G. Intracerebral hemorrhage more than twice as common as subarachnoid hemorrhage. *Journal of Neurosurgery* 1993 ; 78 (2): 188-191.

[29] Kyrosis A, Potagas C, Ghika A, Tsimpouris P.K, Virvidaki E.S, Vemmos K.N. Incidence and predictors of post-stroke aphasia: the arcadia stroke registrery. *The European Journal of Neurology* 2009; 16(6):733-739.

[30] Kumral E, Ozkaya B, Sagduyu A, Sirin H, Vardali E, Pehliva M. The ege stroke registery: a hospital-based study in the aegean region, izmir, Turkey. *Cerebraovscular Diseases.* 8(5): 278-288.

[31] Badjatia N and Rosand J. Intracerebral hemorrhage. *Neurologist* 2005; 14(2): 152-157.

[32] Anderson S.W, Todd M.M, Hindman B.J, Clarke W.R, Torner J.C, Tranel D et al. Effects of intraoperative hypothermia on neuropsychological outcomes after intracranial aneurysm surgery.. *Ann. Neurol.* 2006; 60(5): 518-527.

[33] Helm-Estabrooks N, Albert M.L. Manual of aphasia therapy. 1991. Austin, Texas: Prod-Ed.

[34] Chapey R. ed. Language Intervention Strategies in Aphasia and related Neurogenic Communication disorders. 4th Ed. Baltimore, Maryland: Lippincott Williams and Wilkins; 2001

[35] Isaacs KL, Barr WB, Nelson PK, Devinsky O. Degree of handedness

[36] Knecht S, Dräger B, Deppe M, et al. Handedness and hemispheric language dominance

[37] Mesulam MM. Large-scale neurocognitive networks and distributed processing for attention, language, and memory

[38] Dronkers NF. A new brain

[39] Dronkers NF, Wilkins DP, Van Valin RD Jr, et al. Lesion analysis of the brain

[40] Damasio H, Grabowski TJ, Tranel D, et al. A neural basis for lexical retrieval. *Nature* 1996; 380:499.

[41] Blank SC, Scott SK, Murphy K, et al. Speech production: Wernicke, Broca and beyond. *Brain* 2002; 125:1829.

[42] Hillis AE, Wityk RJ, Barker PB, et al. Subcortical aphasia

[43] Hier D.B, Yoon W.B, Mohr J.P, Price T.R, wolf P.A. Gender and aphasia in the stroke data bank. *Brain and language.* 47(7): 155-167.

[44] Dickey L, Kagan A, Lindsay M.P, Fang J, Rowlan A, Black S. Incidence and profile of inpatient stroke-induced aphasia in Ontario, Canada.. *Archives of Physical Medicine and Rehabilitation* 2010; 91(2): 196-202.

[45] Hilari K: The impact of stroke: are people with aphasia different to those without? *Disabil. Rehabil.* 2011;33(3):211-8.

[46] Stegmayr B, Asplund K, Wester P.O. Trends in incidence , case fatality rate and severity of stroke in northen Sweden, 1985-1991 *Stroke* 1994; 25(9):1738-1745.

[47] Stürmer T, Schlindwein G, Kleiser B, Roemppp A, Brenner H. Clinical diagnosis of ischemic versus hemorrhagic stroke: applicability of existing scores in the emergency situation and proposal of a new score. *Neuroepidemiology* 2002; 21(1):8-17

[48] Bahou Y.G. Intracerebral Hemorrhage. *Neurosciences* 2009; 14(2):152-157.

[49] Tsouli S, Kyritsis A.P, Tsagalis G, Virvidaki E, Vemmos K.N. Signifiance of aphasia first-ever acute stroke: impact on early and late outcome. *Neuroepidemiology* 2009;33(2):96-102.

[50] Bersano A, Burgio F, Gattinoni M, Candelise L. Aphasia burden to hospitalized acute stroke patients: need for an early rehabilitation program.. International journal of stroke: *official journal of the International Stroke Society* 2009; 4(6):443-447.

[51] Urban PP, Wicht S, Vukurevic G et al. Dysarthria in acute ischemic stroke. Lesion topography, clinicoradiologic correlation and etiology. *Neurology* 2001;56:1021-7.

[52] Croquelois A, Bogousslavsky J: Stroke aphasia: 1,500 consecutive cases. *Cerebrovasc. Dis.* 2011;31(4):392-9.

[53] Laska AC, Hellblom A, Murray V, et al.: Aphasia in acute stroke and relation to outcome. *J. Intern. Med.* 2001;249(5):413-22.

[54] Berthier ML: Poststroke aphasia: epidemiology, pathophysiology and treatment. *Drugs Aging* 2005;22(2):163-82.

[55] Black-Schaffer RM, Osberg JS: Return to work after stroke: development of a predictive model. *Arch. Phys. Med. Rehabil.* 1990;71(5):285-90.

[56] Kauhanen ML, Korpelainen JT, Hiltunen P, et al. : Aphasia, depression, and non-verbal cognitive impairment in ischaemic stroke. *Cerebrovasc. Dis.* 2000;10(6):455-61.

[57] Basso A. Prognostic factors in aphasia. *Aphasiology* 1992;1992(6): 337-8.

[58] Maas MB, Lev MH, Ay H, Singhal AB. Greer MD, Smith WS, Harris GJ, Halpern HF,. Koroshetz WJ, and Furie KL; the prognosis for aphasia in stroke. *J. Stroke Cerebrovasc. Dis.* 2010 Dec 23.

[59] Doesborgh SJ, van de Sandt-Koenderman WM, Dippel DW, et al.: Linguistic deficits in the acute phase of stroke. *J. Neurol.* 2003;250(8):977-82.

[60] Code C: Multifactorial processes in recovery from aphasia: developing the foundations for a multileveled framework. *Brain Lang.* 2001;77(1):25-44.

[61] Salter K, Jutai J, Foley N, et al.: Identification of aphasia post stroke: a review of screening assessment tools. *Brain Inj.* 2006;20(6):559-68.

[62] Laska AC, Bartfai A, Hellblom A,et al.: Clinical and prognostic properties of standardized and functional aphasia assessments. *J. Rehabil. Med.* 2007;39:387-392.

[63] Kertesz A. The Western Aphasia Battery. Edited by Grune and Stratton; New York:1982.

[64] Goodglass H, Kaplan E. The Assessment of Aphasia and Related Disorders. 2nd ed. Edited by Lea and Febiger, 2nd, editor. Philadelphia; 1983.

[65] Nicholas LE, Brookshire RH, Macleenan DL, et al.: Revised administration and scoring procedures for the boston naming test and norms for non-brain-damaged adults. *Aphasiology* 1989;3:569-580.

[66] Cote R, Hachinski VC, Shurvell BL, et al.: The canadian neurological scale: A preliminary study in acute stroke. *Stroke* 1986;17:731-737.

[67] Brott T, Adams HP, Jr., Olinger CP, et al.: Measurements of acute cerebral infarction: A clinical examination scale. *Stroke* 1989;20:864-870.

[68] Gotoh F, Terayama Y, Amano T: Development of a novel, weighted, quantifiable stroke scale: Japan stroke scale. *Stroke* 2001;32:1800-1807.

[69] Scandinavian Stroke Study Group: Multicenter trial of hemodilution in ischemic stroke--background and study protocol. *Stroke* 1985;16:885-890.

[70] Adams RJ, Meador KJ, Sethi KD, et al.: Graded neurologic scale for use in acute hemispheric stroke treatment protocols. *Stroke* 1987;18:665-669.

[71] Orgogozo JM, Capildeo R, Anagnostou CN, et al.: Mise au point d'un score neurologique pour l'évaluation clinique des infarctus sylviens. *Presse. Med.* 1983;12:3039-3044.

[72] Crary MA, Haak NJ, Malinsky AE: Preliminary psychometric evaluation of an acute aphasia screening protocol. *Aphasiology* 1989;3:611-618.

[73] Enderby PM, Wood VA, Wade DT, Hewer RL: The frenchay aphasia screening test: A short, simple test for aphasia appropriate for non-specialists. *Int. Rehabil. Med.* 1987;8:166-170.

[74] Nakase-Thompson R, Manning E, Sherer M, et al.: Brief assessment of severe language impairments: Initial validation of the mississippi aphasia screening test. *Brain Inj.* 2005;19:685-691.

[75] Reitan RM, Wolfson D: The halstead-reitan neuropsychological test battery: Theory and clinical interpretation. Tucson: *Neuropsychology Press;* 1985.

[76] Reinvang I, Engvik H: Manual of the norwegian basic aphasia assessement Oslo: Scandinavian University Books; 1980.

[77] Sabe L, Courtis MJ, Saavedra MM, et al.: Desarrollo y validación de una batería corta de evaluación de la afasia : "Bedside de lenguaje". Utilización en un centro de rehabilitación. *Rev. Neurol.* 2008;46:454-460.

[78] Blomert L, Kean ML, Koster C, Scokker J: Amsterdam nijmegen every day langage test: Construction, reliability and validity. *Aphasiology* 1994;8:381-407.

[79] Biniek R, Huber W, Willmes K, et al.: Ein test zur erfassung von sprach- und sprechtstörungen in der akutphase nach schlaganfällen : Aufbau und durchführung. *Nervenarzt* 1991;62:108-115.

[80] Kreisle A, Godefroy O, Delamire C et al. The anatomy of aphasia revisited. *Neurology* 2000;54:1117-123.

[81] Flamand-Roze C, Cauquil-Michon C, Roze E, et al.: Aphasia in border-zone infarcts has a specific initial pattern and good long-term prognosis. *Eur. J. Neurol.* 2011. In press.

[82] Cauquil C, Flamand-Roze C, Denier C: Borderzone Strokes and Transcortical Aphasia. *Curr. Neurol. Neurosci. Rep.* 2011 Sep 9; in press.

[83] Ferreira de Oliveira F, Damasceni BP. A topographic study on the evaluation of speech and language in acute phase of stroke. *Arqu. Neuropsiquiatr.* 2011; 69(5):790-798.

[84] Flamand-Roze C, Falissard B, Roze E, et al.: Validation of a new language screening tool for patients with acute stroke: the Language Screening Test (LAST). *Stroke* 2011;42(5):1224-9.

[85] Kelly H, Brady MC, Enderby P: Speech and language therapy for aphasia following stroke. *Cochrane. Database. Syst. Rev.* 2010;(5):CD000425.

[86] Musso M, Weiller C, Kiebel S, et al.: Training-induced brain plasticity in aphasia. *Brain* 1999;122 (Pt 9):1781-90.

[87] Lazar RM, Minzer B, Antoniello D, et al. : Improvement in aphasia scores after stroke is well predicted by initial severity. *Stroke* 2010;41(7):1485-8.

[88] Kreisel SH, Bazner H, Hennerici MG: Pathophysiology of stroke rehabilitation: temporal aspects of neuro-functional recovery. *Cerebrovasc. Dis.* 2006;21(1-2):6-17.

[89] Berthier ML, Pulvermüller F: Neuroscience insights improve neurorehabilitation of poststroke aphasia. *Nat. Rev. Neurol.* 2011;7(2):86-97.

[90] Saur D, Lange R, Baumgaertner A, et al.: Dynamics of language reorganization after stroke. *Brain* 2006;129(Pt 6):1371-84.

[91] Reineck LA, Agarwal S, Hillis AE: "Diffusion-clinical mismatch" is associated with potential for early recovery of aphasia. *Neurology* 2005;64(5):828-33.

[92] Schlaug G, Marchina S, Norton A: Evidence for plasticity in white-matter tracts of patients with chronic Broca's aphasia undergoing intense intonation-based speech therapy. *Ann. N Y Acad. Sci.* 2009;1169:385-94.

[93] Naeser MA, Palumbo CL: Neuroimaging and language recovery in stroke. *J. Clin. Neurophysiol.* 1994;11(2):150-74.

[94] Winhuisen L, Thiel A, Schumacher B, et al.: Role of the contralateral inferior frontal gyrus in recovery of language function in poststroke aphasia: a combined repetitive transcranial magnetic stimulation and positron emission tomography study. *Stroke* 2005;36(8):1759-63.

[95] Baumgaertner A, Hartwigsen G, Roman Siebner H. Right-heispheric processin of non-linguistic word features: implications for mapping language recovery after stroke. *Hum. Brain Map.* 2012 Feb 22 (ahead of print).

[96] Lidzba k, Staudt M, Zieske F, Schiwilling E, Ackermann H. Prestroke/poststroke fMRI in aphasia: perilesional hemodynamic activation and language recovery. *Neurology* 2012 (78)289-291.

[97] Cicerone KD, Dahlberg C, Malec JF, et al.: Evidence-based cognitive rehabilitation: updated review of the literature from 1998 through 2002. *Arch. Phys. Med. Rehabil.* 2005;86(8):1681-92.

[98] Langhorne P, Bernhardt J, Kwakkel G: Stroke rehabilitation. *Lancet* 2011;377(9778):1693-702.

[99] Cherney, L. R., Patterson, J. P., and Raymer, A. M.: Intensity of aphasia therapy: Evidence and efficacy. *Current Neurology and Neuroscience Reports* 2011, 11(6), 560-569.

[100] Bhogal SK, Teasell R, Speechley M: Intensity of aphasia therapy, impact on recovery. *Stroke* 2003;34(4):987-93.

[101] Hamilton RH, Chrysikou EG, Coslett B: Mechanisms of aphasia recovery after stroke and the role of noninvasive brain stimulation. *Brain Lang*. 2011;118(1-2):40-50.

[102] Dickey, M. W., and Yoo, H.: Predicting outcomes for linguistically specific sentence treatment protocols. *Aphasiology* 2010, 24(6-8), 787-801.

[103] Godecke E, Hird K, Lalor EE, Rai T, et al.: Very early poststroke aphasia therapy: a pilot randomized controlled efficacy trial. *Int. J. Stroke* 2011 Oct 6; in press.

[104] Sarkamo T, Tervaniemi M, Laitinen S, et al. : Music listening enhances cognitive recovery and mood after middle cerebral artery stroke. *Brain* 2008;131(Pt 3):866-76.

[105] Conklyn D, Novak E, Boissy A, Berthoux F, Chemali K. The effects of Modified Melodic Intonation Therapy on Non fluent aphasia- A pilot study. *J. Speech Lang. Hear. Res.* 2012 March (ahead of print).

[106] Simmons-Mackie, N., Raymer, A., Armstrong, E., Holland, A., and Cherney, L. R.: Communication partner training in aphasia: A systematic review. *Archives of Physical Medicine and Rehabilitation* 2010:91(12), 1814-1837.

[107] Laska AC, Kahan T, Hellblom A, et al.: A randomized controlled trial on very early speech and language therapy in acute stroke patients with aphasia. *Cerebrovascular Disease* 2011:in press.

[108] Marshall RC: The impact of intensity of aphasia therapy on recovery. *Stroke* 2008;39(2):e48.

In: Aphasia   ISBN: 978-1-62257-681-4
Editors: E. Holmgren, E.S. Rudkilde   © 2013 Nova Science Publishers, Inc.

Chapter V

A New Classification of Aphasias

*Alfredo Ardila**
Department of Communication Sciences and Disorders
Florida International University, Miami, FL, US

Abstract

In this chapter it is emphasized that there are only two fundamental forms of aphasia, which are linked to impairments in the lexical/semantic and grammatical systems of language (Wernicke-type aphasia and Broca-type aphasia, respectively). Other aphasic syndromes do not really impair language knowledge per se, but rather either some peripheral mechanisms required to produce language (conduction aphasia and aphasia of the supplementary motor area), or the executive control of the language (extra-Sylvian or transcortical motor aphasia). A new classification of aphasic syndromes is suggested. In this proposed classification a distinction is established between primary (or ''central'') aphasias (Wernicke's aphasia—three subtypes—and Broca's aphasia); secondary (or ''peripheral'') aphasias (conduction aphasia and supplementary motor area aphasia); and dysexecutive aphasia.

* 11200 SW 8th Street, AHC3-431B; Florida International University; Miami, Florida 33199; Email: ardilla@fiu.edu.

Introduction

Aphasia represents the most studied cognitive syndrome associated with brain pathology. As a matter of fact, the analysis of aphasia represents the initial question and departing point in modern cognitive neuroscience. Understanding aphasia is consequently most crucial in our interpretations about brain organization of cognition.

Diverse aphasia classifications have been proposed since Broca's first description of a language disturbance associated with brain pathology (Broca, 1863). There are, however, two most influential aphasia classifications, that have significantly guided the area during the last decades: the Boston Group classification (Geschwind, Benson, Alexander, Goodglass, Kaplan, and others); and Luria's aphasia interpretation. The first one has been particularly influential in the US and western European countries; the second one has been mostly used in eastern European countries and Latin America.

Boston Group classification represents a further development of Wernicke's ideas about brain organization of language, and includes two basic distinctions: (1) aphasias can be fluent or non-fluent; and (2) aphasias can be cortical, subcortical, or transcortical (e.g., Albert, Goodglass, Helm, Rubers, & Alexander, 1981; Alexander & Benson, 1991; Benson, 1979; Benson & Geschwind, 1971, 1985; Geschwind, 1965; Goodglass, 1993; Goodglass & Kaplan, 1972). Conduction aphasia (initially proposed by Wernicke in 1874 and described by Lichtheim in 1885) was introduced to account for the language repetition impairments frequently found in left parietal (or insular) damage.

Luria (1966, 1970, 1974, 1976, 1980) proposed, initially six, but later seven aphasia subtypes: motor efferent or kinetic, motor afferent or kinesthetic, acoustic-agnosic, acoustic-amnesic, amnesic, semantic, and dynamic). Luria assumed that in each aphasia subtype there is a particular language processing defect. In Luria's approach, aphasia subtypes and names refer to the specific level of language that is impaired.

Benson and Ardila (1996) attempted to integrate both points of view and proposed a classification based on two different anatomical criteria: (1) aphasia can be pre-Rolandic (anterior, non-fluent) or post-Rolandic (posterior, fluent); and (2) aphasia can be associated with pathology in the peri- Sylvian language area (peri-Sylvian aphasias); or aphasia is due to damage beyond this area (extra-Sylvian). Subtypes were introduced for some aphasia syndromes. Aphasias were also regarded as anatomical syndromes

(Table 1). This classification is currently used by different authors (e.g., Basso, 2003).

Table 1. Two major parameters are used in aphasia classification: (a) Aphasia can be pre-Rolandic or post-Rolandic; (b) Aphasia can be peri-Sylvian or extra-Sylvian. Clinical syndromes are related to anatomical syndromes

	Pre-Rolandic	Post-Rolandic
Peri-	Broca's Type I	Conduction
Sylvian	(triangular syndrome)	(parietal-insular syndrome)
	Broca's Type II	Wernicke's Type I
	(triangular-opercular-syndrome)	(posterior insular-temporal isthmus syndrome)
		Wernicke's Type II (superior and middle temporal gyrus syndrome)
Extra-Sylvian	Extra-Sylvian Motor Type I (left prefrontal dorsolateral syndrome)	Extra-Sylvian Sensory Type I (temporal-occipital syndrome)
	Extra-Sylvian Motor Type II (supplementary motor area syndrome)	Extra-Sylvian Sensory Type II (parieto-occipital angular syndrome)

According to Benson & Ardila, 1996.

During the last decades significant advances in the understanding of brain organization of language has been obtained. Contemporary neuroimaging techniques, such as fMRI (e.g., Meinzer, Harnish, Conway & Crosson, 2011; Zahn et al., 2000), PET (Cao, George, Ewing, Vikingstad & Johnson, 1998) and tractography (Song et al., 2011; Yamada et al., 2007), have significantly extended our understanding of the organization of language in the brain under normal and abnormal conditions (Lee, Kannan & Hillis, 2006; Small & Burton, 2002); a significantly better understanding of the brain circuitries supporting language has been developed (e.g., Ullman, 2004); and a re-analysis of the classical language areas (Broca's and Wernicke's) has been developed (e.g., Grodzinky & Amunts, 2006); and new scientific discoveries, such as the "mirror neurons", have changed our understanding of the functioning of the human brain, including language organization (e.g., Rizzolati & Arbib, 1998). In this chapter a further attempt is made to integrate these new advances; a new classification of aphasia syndromes will be proposed. This new aphasia classification was recently presented (Ardila, 2010) and has been discussed by several authors (e.g., Buckingham, 2010; Kertesz, 2010; Marshall, 2010).

There Are Only Two Major Aphasic Syndromes

There is a fundamental point in the analysis of aphasia: aphasia is not one, but two different clinical syndromes, initially described by Broca in 1861 and Wernicke in 1874. These two syndromes have been named in different ways, but roughly corresponding to Wernicke-type aphasia and Broca-type aphasia (e.g., Ardila, 2010; Albert et al., 1981; Alexander & Benson, 1991; Bastian, 1898; Benson & Ardila, 1996; Freud, 1891/1973; Goldstein, 1948; Head, 1926; Hecaen, 1972; Kertesz, 1979; Lichtheim, 1885; Luria, 1976; Pick, 1931; Schuell, Jenkins, & Jimenez-Pabon, 1964; Taylor-Sarno, 1998; Wilson, 1926; see Tesak & Code, 2008, for review).

Aphasia represents a language disturbance and consequently, not only a neurologic/anatomic but also a linguistic understanding is required. Jakobson (1964; Jakobson & Halle, 1956) proposed that these two major aphasic syndromes are related to the two basic linguistic operations: selecting (language as paradigm) and sequencing (language as syntagm). Jakobson (1964) proposed that aphasia tends to involve one of two types of linguistic deficiency. A patient may lose the ability to use language in two rather different ways: the language impairment can be situated on the paradigmatic axis (similarity disorder) or the syntagmatic axis (contiguity disorder). The first one is related with the Wernicke-type aphasia, and the second one with the Broca-type aphasia.

Wernicke-Type Aphasia

In Wernicke-type aphasia the lexical repertoire tends to decrease and language-understanding difficulties are evident. Wernicke's aphasia patients may not fully discriminate the acoustic information contained in speech (Robson, Keidel, Ralph & Sage, 2012). Lexical (words) and semantic (meanings) associations become deficient. In Wernicke-type aphasia the language defect is situated at the level of meaningful words (nouns). Phoneme and word selection are deficient, but language syntax (contiguity:

sequencing elements) is well preserved and even overused (paragrammatism in Wernicke aphasia). Wernicke-type aphasia represents the clinical syndrome characterized by impairments in the selection process (paradigmatic axis defect). Patients with Wernicke aphasia have problems in recalling the words (memory of the words) and also in associating the words with specific meanings: the semantics of the words can be abnormal. This means that at least three different deficits underlie Wernicke-type aphasia: (1) phoneme discrimination impairments (auditory verbal agnosia); (2) verbal memory impairments; and finally (3) lexical/semantic association deficits. Robson, Sage and Ralph (2012) emphasized that deficits responsible for the comprehension defects in Wernicke aphasia are diverse, including acoustic-phonological defects, and semantic deficits.

Figure 1 presents in a summarized form the model proposed by Ardila (1993) to account for language recognition. It is assumed that there are three different levels of language understanding (phoneme recognition, lexical recognition, and semantic recognition). These three language understanding levels can be impaired in cases of Wernicke-type of aphasia. In consequence, there are three different subtypes of Wernicke aphasia: Acoustic-agnosic type (associated with phoneme recognition defects), acoustic amnesic type (associated with lexical recognition defects), and amnesic, nominal or traditionally called transcortical (extrasylvian) sensory aphasia (associated with semantic recognition defects).

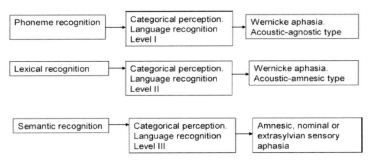

Adapted from Ardila, 1993.

Figure 1. Three levels of language recognition potentially impaired in Wernicke-type aphasia can be distinguished: phonemic (categorical perception level I), lexical (categorical perception level II), and semantic (categorical perception level III). Three different sub-syndromes can be found: phonemic discrimination defects (acoustic-agnosic or Wernicke's aphasia type I), verbal-acoustic memory defects (acoustic-amnesic or Wernicke's aphasia type II), and semantic association defects (amnesic, nominal or extra-Sylvian sensory aphasia).

Broca-Type Aphasia

In Broca-type of aphasia, language defects are quite different; while the lexical/semantic dimension of the language is preserved, grammar is seriously impaired.

Language is scarce, nonfluent, and poorly articulated, but language understanding is relatively well preserved. That means, the selection process (paradigmatic axis) is normal.According to Jakobson (1964) in Broca-type aphasia the syntagmatic axis of language is impaired. There is a defect in language sequencing (morphosyntax).

Indeed, in Broca's aphasia two different distinguishing characteristics can be observed, one at the motor level and the other at the purely language level: (1) there is on one hand a motor component (lack of fluency, disintegration of the speech kinetic melodies, verbal-articulatory impairments, etc., that is usually referred as apraxia of speech); and (2) on the other hand, there is a reduction in the grammar, usually referred as agrammatism (e.g., Benson & Ardila, 1996; Berndt & Caramazza, 1980; Goodglass, 1993; Kertesz, 1985; Luria, 1976). Interestingly, a large part of the fronto-parieto-temporal cortex has been observed to be involved with syntactic-morphological functions (Bhatnagar, Mandybur, Buckingham, & Andy, 2000).

Apraxia of speech has been observed specifically associated with damage in the left precentral gyrus of the insula (Dronkers, 1996; but see Hillis et al., 2004) It should be noted that not all of apraxia of speech is indeed a contiguity disorder; there are many phonetic-level errors in apraxia of speech that have more to do with segmental distortions. If both impairments (apraxia of speech and agrammatism) are simultaneously observed (i.e., they are very highly correlated), it can be assumed they are just two different manifestations of a single underlying defect. It is not easy to understand which one could be the single factor responsible for these two clinical manifestations, but it may be kind of "inability to sequence expressive elements". Broca's area, most likely, is not specialized in producing language, but in certain neural activity that can support not only skilled movements required for speech, but also morphosyntax. It has been observed that indeed language networks supporting grammar and fluency are overlapped in the brain (Borovsky, Saygin, Bates, & Dronkers, 2007).

How to Interpret Other Aphasic Disturbances?

Frequently it has been assumed that three major (perisylvian) aphasic syndromes can be distinguished: frontal Broca aphasia, temporal Wernicke aphasia, and parietal conduction aphasia (e.g., Benson, 1979; Goodglass, 1993). These are the three aphasia disorders associated with damage in the so-called "brain language area"; a concept introduced by Dejerine (1914), roughly corresponding to the perisylvian area of the left hemisphere, and including partially the frontal, temporal and parietal lobes of the left hemisphere.

In addition to Broca, Wernicke and conduction aphasia, aphasia classifications generally include a diversity of additional language disturbances, such as transcortical (extra-Sylvian) aphasia, and anomic aphasia (e.g., Alexander & Benson, 1991; Benson & Geschwind, 1971; Hecaen & Albert, 1978; Kertesz, 1979; Lecours, Lhermitte, & Bryans, 1983; Luria, 1966). However, some aphasic syndromes can eventually be considered as variants of the Broca and Wernicke aphasias. For instance, as mentioned above, amnesic or anomic or nominal aphasia (usually due to damage in the vicinity of BA 37) (Head, 1926; Hecaen & Albert, 1978; Luria, 1976), as well as transcortical sensory aphasia can be interpreted as subtypes of Wernicke aphasia in which the semantic associations of the words are significantly impaired (see Figure 1).

No question, the major difficulty in interpreting these additional syndromes refers to conduction aphasia, considering that conduction aphasia is frequently regarded as one out the three major aphasia syndromes (in addition to Broca aphasia and Wernicke aphasia).

Conduction Aphasia

A crucial question is, how conduction aphasia—a well recognized and extensively studied aphasic syndrome (e.g., Benson & Ardila, 1994; Damasio & Damasio, 1980; Goldstein, 1948; Kohn, 1992) — can be interpreted?

The most frequent, and classic, explanation of conduction aphasia is as a disconnection syndrome (e.g., Damasio & Damasio 1980; Geschwind 1965; Wernicke 1874), usually due to a lesion affecting the arcuate fasciculus (Yamada et al., 2007) and sporadically an indirect pathway passing through the inferior parietal cortex (Catani, Jones, & Ffytche, 2005). This is the usually explanation, sometimes referred as the Wernicke-Geschwind disconnection model of conduction aphasia. Alternatively, conduction aphasia has also been interpreted as a segmentary ideomotor apraxia (e.g., Ardila & Rosselli., 1990; Brown, 1972, 1975; Luria 1976, 1980). According to this second interpretation, conduction aphasia could be regarded as a verbal apraxia, an ideomotor apraxia impairing the movements required for speaking, or simply as a kinesthetic apraxia of speech. Luria (1976) suggested that paraphasias in conduction aphasia (Luria's kinesthetic motor or afferent motor aphasia) are indeed articulatory-based deviations (articulatory literal paraphasias), not really phonological disturbances. Paraphasias in conduction aphasia are due mainly to phoneme substitutions and phoneme deletions; they result basically in switches in phoneme manner and place of articulation (Ardila, 1992). Similarities between errors in ideomotor apraxia and conduction aphasia language deficits have been suggested.

According to Benson, Sheretaman, Bouchard, Segarra, Price, and Geschwind (1973) conduction aphasia has three fundamental and five secondary characteristics; so-called secondary characteristics are frequently but not necessarily found in conduction aphasia. The three basic characteristics are: (1) fluent conversational language; (2) comprehension almost normal; and (3) significant impairments in repetition. Secondary characteristics include: (1) impairments in naming; (2) reading impairments; (3) variable writing difficulties (apraxic agraphia); (4) ideomotor apraxia; and (5) additional neurological impairments. Bartha and Benke (2003) report that conduction aphasia patients present as relatively homogenic in their aphasic manifestations: severe impairment of repetition and fluent expressive language functions with frequent phonemic paraphasias, repetitive self-corrections, word-finding difficulties, and paraphrasing. Repetitive self-corrections frequently result in so-called *conduit d'approche*. Language comprehension (auditory and reading) is only mildly impaired.

Benson et al.'s. (1973) description of conduction aphasia clearly recognizes that spontaneous language production and language understanding are significantly preserved. In consequence, some mechanisms required for correct language repetition are impaired, but the knowledge of language itself (phonology, lexicon, semantics, and grammar) is not impaired. The critical question is: Should conduction aphasia be interpreted as a primary aphasic syndrome? Indeed, language repetition impairments can be observed in different aphasia syndromes and language repetition has also been interpreted as a right hemisphere ability (Berthier et al., 1991).

The distinction between "aphasias with repetition impairments" vs "aphasias without repetition impairments" is indeed a general and crude distinction. It has been proposed that different aphasia groups (including the so-called transcortical aphasias) may present language repetition errors; but depending on the specific repetition task, errors may be evident or may be unnoticed in a particular aphasic group (Ardila & Rosselli, 1992). Different mechanisms underlying repetition deficits have been proposed: limitation of auditory-verbal short-term memory, difficulties at the level of phonological production, impairments in phoneme recognition, and semantic and syntactic comprehension defects. Simply speaking, different deficits can be responsible for the repetition defects found in aphasia. Furthermore, difficulties in language repetition depend on the specific repetition task (short words, long sentences, meaningful, meaningless, etc).

Conduction aphasia is, consequently, not a primary form of aphasia, but rather a secondary (or "peripheral") defect in language indirectly affecting a specific language ability (i.e., the ability to repeat). Language itself is not impaired, but rather it represents an impaired ability to reproduce aloud the auditory information that is heard.

Of course, this is an important skill used not only to develop language but also to use it correctly. Interpreting conduction aphasia as a secondary (or "peripheral") defect in language (rather than a primary or central form of aphasia) does not in any way decrease the importance of repetition in language.

In brief, it can be argued that conduction aphasia can be interpreted as a "secondary" (or "peripheral") language disturbance, rather than a primary (or "central") form of aphasia. Language knowledge is well preserved in conduction aphasia, but there is a limitation in a particular language function, i.e., repetition. Obviously, if some animals can repeat, that means that language repetition cannot be considered as a primary linguistic ability.

Interestingly, Jakobson (1964) suggested a similar distinction when proposing that in aphasia language could be either "disintegrated" or "limited" (disintegration vs limitation in aphasia).

Obviously language is disintegrated only in Wernicke and Broca aphasia. In other forms of aphasia, including conduction aphasia, language is limited, not disintegrated.

Transcortical (Extra-Sylvian) Motor Aphasia

Patients with left convexital prefrontal damage usually present a lack of verbal initiative and a significant limitation in the active use of the language, referred as transcortical (extra-Sylvian) or dynamic aphasia. Extra-Sylvian (transcortical) motor aphasia could be interpreted as an executive function defect specifically affecting language use. The ability to actively and appropriately generate language appears impaired while the phonology, lexicon, semantics, and grammar are preserved.

Should the ability to correctly generate language be regarded as a linguistic ability (i.e., cognitive ability)? Or rather, should it be considered as an executive function ability (i.e., metacognitive ability)? It does not seem difficult to argue that the ability to correctly organize language sequences can be regarded as an executive function and as a metacognitive ability rather than a purely linguistic ability. Some rationales to support this interpretation are: (1) It could be argued that in extra-Sylvian (transcortical) motor aphasia there is a defect in verbal initiative rather than in language knowledge (Kleist, 1934). (2) Different authors (for example, Luria, 1976, 1980) have emphasized that this type of aphasia shares the general characteristics of prefrontal (i.e., dysexecutive) syndrome but specifically with regard to verbal processes. This means, it is the prefrontal (dysexecutive) syndrome affecting the verbal processes (Gold et al., 1997). (3) Further, the impairment in extra-Sylvian (transcortical) motor aphasia does not affect language understanding, and fundamental linguistic processes are preserved (Berthier, 1999). And finally, (4) it could be argued that the prefrontal cortex does not participate in basic cognition, but rather in metacognition (e.g., Ardila & Surloff, 2011).

In consequence, extra-Sylvian (transcortical) motor aphasia does not necessarily have to be interpreted as a primary aphasic syndrome, but rather as a language disturbance due to a more general intellectual impairment (dysexecutive syndrome). Extra-Sylvian (transcortical) motor aphasia could indeed be referred to as "dysexecutive aphasia". Some authors have previously interpreted extra-Sylvian motor aphasia in a similar way (e.g., Luria 1976, 1980). Alexander (2006) suggested that transcortical motor aphasia could be more accurately defined as an executive function disorder rather than aphasia. He proposed that the progression of clinical disorders from aphasia to discourse impairments can be interpreted as a sequence of procedural impairments from basic morpho-syntax to elaborated grammar to narrative language, correlated with a progression of the focus of the damage from posterior frontal to polar and/or lateral frontal to medial frontal.

Transcortical (Extra-Sylvian) Sensory Aphasia

Transcortical (extra-Sylvian) sensory aphasia (TSA) has been a polemic syndrome. Seemingly, the polemic is related to the way TSA is defined.

TSA has been defined in two partially different ways; (1) according to its "basic" definition, TSA is a fluent language disorder characterized by impaired auditory comprehension, with preserved repetition (Albert et al., 1981; Berthier, 1999; Goldstein, 1948; Lichtheim, 1885). Consequently, there are only three distinguishing characteristics in TSA (normal fluency, impaired auditory comprehension, and preserved repetition). In such a case, TSA presents similar deficits as in Wernicke's aphasia, but repetition ability is spared and phoneme discrimination impairments are not found. (2) According to its "extended" definition, TSA also includes a semantic jargon (Goodglass, 1993; Kertesz, 1982; Lecours, Osborn, Travies, Rouillon, & Lavalle-Huyng, 1981). Kertesz (1985, p. 317) makes a comprehensive definition of TSA: "TSA is characterized by fluent and often irrelevant speech output, very poor comprehension and well-preserved repetition. Spontaneous speech often consists of semantic jargon that has no relationship to what is being asked of the patient". This definition clearly recognizes that there are three basic characteristics, and sometimes jargon is found. But jargon is not a required symptom for the diagnosis of TSA. By the same token, other language impairments can also be found, such as poor naming, and preserved oral reading with impaired reading comprehension, but their presence is not essential to establish the diagnosis of TSA (Berthier, 1999).

According to Berthier (1999) the most common pattern of verbal expression is represented by the so-called "semantic" or "verbal" jargon (e.g., Lecours & Rouillon, 1976). There is an abundant language production, with reduction of meaningful words conferring the impression of emptiness. The content of the sentence is irrelevant. Furthermore, TSA patients appear unaware of their logorrhea (Lebrun, 1987). A second pattern of spontaneous speech described by Berthier (1999) is referred to as "anomic" and is associated with an impaired access to content words. This second pattern corresponds to the TSA "basic" definition mentioned above.

Because repetition is spared, phonological processing is assumed to be preserved, at least partially, while lexical-semantic information included in the word meaning is impaired (Boatman et al., 2000). Usually, it is accepted that TSA is associated with relatively extensive posterior lesions including the temporo-parieto-occipital junction of the left hemisphere but sparing the areas around the primary auditory cortex (Berthier, 1999). Damasio (1991) observed that TSA is associated with lesions involving the temporal-occipital area (BA 37), the angular gyrus (BA 39), or the white matter underlying these regions, but sparing the primary auditory cortex (BA 41 and 42), and BA 22. Damasio suggested that the core area for TSA is the temporal-occipital area (BA 37) with variable extension to the occipital lobe and the angular gyrus. Kertesz (1982) analyzed 15 patients with TSA and proposed two different subgroups: one is more medial, inferior, and posterior and is clearly in the posterior cerebral artery territory; and the other is relatively more lateral, superior, and anterior and seems to be in a watershed area between middle cerebral and posterior cerebral arteries.

Benson and Ardila (1996), considering this variability in TSA, also distinguished two subtypes: the first one similar to Luria's amnesic aphasia (BA 37), and the second one corresponding Luria's semantic aphasia (BA 39). This distinction is coincidental with the neuroanatomical correlates of TSA found by Damasio (1991).

Recent reports support the assumption that TSA is usually found associated with extensive lesions of the left hemisphere (e.g., Warabi, Bandoh, Kurisaki, Nishio, & Hayashi, 2006), generally involving large portions of the temporal-parietal-occipital areas. According to Alexander, Hiltbrunner, and Fischer (1989) the critical lesion for transcortical sensory aphasia in these patients involved pathways in the posterior periventricular white matter adjacent to the posterior temporal isthmus, pathways that are most likely converging on the inferolateral temporo-occipital cortex.

TSA represents a disorder in the semantic recognition of language that may or may not be associated during the acute stage with other language impairments, specially logorrhea and jargon, depending on the extension of the lesion. But logorrhea and jargon are not required in the definition of TSA.

Supplementary Motor Area (SMA) Aphasia

This is a type of language disturbance recognized relative late in the aphasia history. Supplementary motor area (SMA) aphasia indeed is not associated with damage in the so-called "language area" of the brain. Penfield and Welch (1951) first observed arrest of speech associated with stimulation of this cortical region. Clinical characteristics of this type of aphasia were described by Rubens (1975, 1976).

Language disturbances in cases of damage of the left SMA have been characterized by, (1) an initial mutism lasting about 2–10 days; (2) later, a virtually total inability to initiate speech, (3) a nearly normal speech repetition, (4) a normal language understanding, and (5) absence of echolalia. A right leg paresis and right leg sensory loss are observed; a mild right shoulder paresis and Babinski sign are also found. Language recovery is outstanding and it is usually observed during the following few weeks or months (Ardila & Benson, 1996; Rubens, 1975, 1976). The occlusion of the left anterior cerebral artery is the most frequent etiology, but it has also been reported in cases of tumors and traumatic head injury (e.g., Ardila & Lopez, 1984).

SMA is a premotor area (medial extension of BA 6) participating in initiating, maintaining, coordinating, and planning complex sequences of movements; it receives information from the posterior parietal and frontal association areas, and projects to the primary motor cortex (Kandel, Schwartz & Jessell, 1995). SMA damage is also associated with slow reaction time (Alexander, Stuss, Picton, Shallice, & Gillingham, 2007). It has been observed that activation of the SMA precedes voluntary movement (Erdler et al., 2000); a crucial role in the motor expression of speech processing has also been postulated (Fried et al., 1991). Nonetheless, the SMA is located some distance -and indeed far away- from the classic language area postulated by Dejerine (1914) and assumed in most anatomical models of aphasia. Neuroimaging studies in humans have demonstrated that SMA is active when performing various cognitive tasks, such as spatial working memory (Jonides et al., 1993), verbal working memory (Paulesu, Frith, & Frackowiak, 1993), arithmetic tasks (Dehaene et al., 1996; Hanakawa et al., 2002), spatial mental imagery (Mellet et al., 1996), and spatial attention (Simon et al., 2002).

Evidently, the SMA is a complex motor cortical area, not primarily a language related brain area. Its role in language seemingly refers to the motor ability to initiate and maintain voluntary speech production.

Conclusion

From the above analysis it is evident that the term ''aphasia'' has been used to refer both to primary language disturbances, affecting the language system itself (phonology, lexicon, semantics, grammar), and to other impairments not affecting the language system itself, but affecting some abilities required for using language. Aphasia is usually interpreted and understood as a disturbance in the language, not in some mechanisms required to produce and use the language. A major distinction can be established between primary language disturbances (central aphasias, language is disintegrated), and secondary language disturbances resulting from "peripheral" impairments (secondary or "peripheral" aphasias; language is limited). In the primary aphasia the language itself is impaired. In the secondary language disturbances, some mechanism required to produce the language is altered. Sometimes language is not impaired, but the patient cannot use it appropriately because of executive control impairments (dysexecutive aphasia).

Table 2 presents a proposed interpretation and classification of aphasia syndromes. A distinction between primary aphasias (Wernicke-type and Broca-type; language is disintegrated as a paradigm --selection process--; or as a syntagm --sequencing process--) and secondary aphasias (conduction aphasia and aphasia of the supplementary motor area; language is limited in a specific aspect) is introduced; extra-Sylvian (or transcortical) motor aphasia is interpreted as a dysexecutive aphasia (the active use and executive control of the language is limited).

Table 2. A proposed new classification of aphasias. A distinction between primary aphasias (Wernicke-type and Broca-type) and secondary aphasias (conduction aphasia and aphasia of the supplementary motor area) is introduced; extra-Sylvian (or transcortical) motor aphasia is interpreted as a dysexecutive aphasia

Type	Impairment
Primary (central) aphasias	*Language system impaired*
Wernicke-type aphasia (fluent aphasia)	Phonological level
	Lexical level
	Semantic level
Broca-type aphasia(non-fluent aphasia)	Sequencing expressive elements at syntactic and phonetic level
Secondary (peripheral) aphasias	*Mechanisms of production impaired*
Conduction aphasia	Disconnection (or segmentary ideamotora verbal apraxia)
SMA aphasia	To initiate and maintain voluntary speech production
Dysexecutive aphasia	*Language executive control impaired*
Extra-Sylvian (transcortical) motor aphasia	Executive control of language

According to Ardila, 2010.

References

Albert, M. L., Goodglass, H., Helm, N. A., Rubers, A. B., & Alexander, M. P. (1981). *Clinical aspects of dysphasia.* New York: Springer-Verlag.

Alexander, M. P. (2006). Impairments of procedures for implementing complex language are due to disruption of frontal attention processes. *Journal of the International Neuropsychological Society*, 12, 236–247.

Alexander, M. P., & Benson, D. F. (1991). The aphasia and related disturbances. In R. J. Joynt (Ed.), *Clinical neurology* (pp. 1–58). Philadelphia: Lippincott.

Alexander, M. P., Hiltbrunner, B., & Fischer, R. S. (1989). Distributed anatomy of transcortical sensory aphasia. *Archives of Neurology*, 46, 885–892.

Alexander, M. P., Stuss, D. T., Picton, T., Shallice, T., & Gillingham, S. (2007). Regional frontal injuries cause distinct impairments in cognitive control. *Neurology*, 68, 1515–1523.

Ardila, A. (1992). Phonological transformations in conduction aphasia. *Journal of Psycholinguistic Research*, 21, 473–484.

Ardila, A. (1993). Toward a model of phoneme perception. *International Journal of Neuroscience*, 70, 1–12.

Ardila, A. (2010). A proposed reinterpretation and reclassification of aphasia syndromes. *Aphasiology.* 24 (3), 363–394

Ardila, A., & Lopez, M. V. (1984). Transcortical motor aphasia: One or two aphasias? *Brain and Language*, 22, 350–353.

Ardila, A., & Rosselli, M. (1990). Conduction aphasia and verbal apraxia. *Journal of Neurolinguistics*, 5, 1–14.

Ardila, A., & Rosselli, M. (1992). Repetition in aphasia. *Journal of Neurolinguistics*, 7, 103–133.

Ardila, A., & Surloff, C. (2011). *Executive dysfunction.* In S. Gilman (Ed.) Medlink Neurology. San Diego,CA: Arbor Publishing.

Bartha, L., & Benke, T. (2003). Acute conduction aphasia: An analysis of 20 cases. *Brain and Language*, 85, 93–108.

Basso, A. (2003). *Aphasia and its therapy.* New York: Oxford University Press.

Bastian, D. C. (1898). *Aphasia and other speech defects.* London: H. K. Lewis.

Benson, D. F. (1979). *Aphasia, alexia and agraphia.* New York: Churchill Livingstone.

Benson, D. F., & Ardila, A. (1994). Conduction aphasia: A syndrome of language network disruption. In H. Kirshner (Ed.), *Handbook of speech and language disorders*. New York: Mercel Dekker Inc.

Benson, D. F., & Ardila, A. (1996). *Aphasia: A clinical perspective*. New York: Oxford University Press.

Benson, D. F., & Geschwind, N. (1971). Aphasia and related cortical disturbances. In A. B. Baker & L. H. Baker (Eds.), *Clinical neurology*. Philadelphia: Harper & Row.

Benson, D. F., & Geschwind, N. (1985). The aphasia and related disturbances. In A. B. Baker & R. J. Joynt (Eds.), *Clinical neurology*. Philadelphia: Harper & Row.

Benson, D. F., Sheretaman, W. A., Bouchard, R., Segarra, J. M., Price, D., & Geschwind, N. (1973). Conduction aphasia: A clinicopathological study. *Archives of Neurology*, 28, 339–346.

Berndt, R. S., & Caramazza, A. (1980). A redefinition of the syndrome of Broca's aphasia: Implications for a neuropsychological model of language. *Applied Psycholinguistics*, 1, 225–278.

Berthier, M. (1999). *Transcortical aphasias*. Hove, UK: Psychology Press.

Berthier, M. L., Starkstein, S. E., Leiguarda, R., Ruiz, A., Mayberg, H. S., & Wagner, H. et al. (1991). Transcortical aphasia. Importance of the nonspeech dominant hemisphere in language repetition. *Brain*, 114, 1409–1427.

Bhatnagar, S. C., Mandybur, G. T., Buckingham, H. W., & Andy, O. J. (2000). Language representation in the human brain: Evidence from cortical mapping. *Brain and Language*, 74, 238–259.

Boatman, D., Gordon, B., Hart, J., Selnes, O., Miglioretti, D., & Lenz, F. (2000). Transcortical sensory aphasia: Revisited and revised. *Brain*, 123, 1634–1642.

Borovsky, A., Saygin, A. P., Bates, E., & Dronkers, N. (2007). Lesion correlates of conversational speech production deficits. *Neuropsychologia*, 45, 2525–2533.

Broca, P. (1863). Localisation des fonctions ce´re´brales: Siege du langage articule´. *Bulletin de la Societe´ d'Anthropologie*, 4, 200–203.

Brown, J. W. (1972). *Aphasia, agnosia and apraxia*. Springfield, IL: Thomas.

Brown, J. M. (1975). The problem of repetition: A case study of conduction aphasia and the 'isolation' syndrome. *Cortex*, 11, 37–52.

Buckingham, H.W. (2010). Aristotle's functional association psychology. The syntagmatic and the paradigmatic axes in the neurolinguistics of

Roman Jakobson and Alexander Luria: An anatomical and functional quagmire. *Aphasiology.* 24 (3), 395-403.

Cao, Y., George, K. P., Ewing, J. R., Vikingstad, E. M., & Johnson, A. F. (1998). Neuroimaging of language and aphasia after stroke. *Journal of Cerebrovascular Diseases,* 7, 230–233.

Catani, M., Jones, D. K., & Ffytche, D. H. (2005). Perisylvian language networks of the human brain. *Annals of Neurology*, 57, 8–16.

Damasio, H. (1991). Neuroanatomical correlates of the aphasias. In M. Taylor Sarno (Ed.), *Acquired aphasia* (pp. 45–71). New York: Academic Press.

Damasio, H., & Damasio, A. (1980). The anatomical basis of conduction aphasia. *Brain,* 103, 337–350.

Dehaene, S., Tzourio, N., Frak, V., Raynaud, L., Cohen, L., & Mehler, J. et al. (1996). Cerebral activations during number multiplication and comparison: A PET study. *Neuropsychologia*, 34, 1097–1106.

Dejerine, J. (1914). Semiologie des affections du systeme nerveux. Paris: Masson.

Erdler, M., Beisteiner, R., Mayer, D., Kaindl, T., Edward, V., & Windischberger, C. et al. (2000). Supplementary motor area activation preceding voluntary movement is detectable with a whole-scalp magnetoencephalography system. *Neuroimage*, 11, 697–670.

Freud, S. (1891/1973*). Las afasias.* Buenos Aires: Ediciones Nueva Vision.

Fried, I., Katz, A., McCarthy, G., Sass, K. J., Williamson, P., & Spencer, S. S. et al. (1991). Functional organisation of human supplementary motor cortex studied by electrical stimulation. *Journal of Neurosciences*, 11, 3656–3666.

Geschwind, N. (1965). Disconnection syndromes in animals and man. *Brain*, 88, 237–294.

Gold, M., Nadeau, S. E., Jacobs, D. H., Adair, J. C., Rothi, L. J., & Heilman, K. M. (1997). Adynamic aphasia: A transcortical motor aphasia with defective semantic strategy formation. *Brain and Language*, 57, 374–393.

Goldstein, K. (1948). *Language and language disturbances*. New York: Grune & Stratton.

Goodglass, H. (1993). *Understanding aphasia*. New York: Academic Press.

Goodglass, H., & Kaplan, E. (1972). *The assessment of aphasia and related disorders*. Philadelphia: Lea & Febiger.

Grodzinky, Y., & Amunts, K. (Eds.). (2006). *Broca's region*. New York: Oxford University Press.

Hanakawa, T., Hondam, M., Sawamoto, N., Okada, T., Yonekura, Y., & Fukuyama, H. et al. (2002). The role of rostral Brodmann area 6 in mental-operation tasks: An integrative neuroimaging approach. *Cerebral Cortex*, 12, 1157–1170.

Head, H. (1926). *Aphasia and kindred disorders of speech*. London: Cambridge University Press.

Hecaen, H. (1972). *Introduction a la neuropsychologie*. Paris: Larousse.

Hecaen, H., & Albert, M. L. (1978). *Human neuropsychology*. New York: Wiley.

Hillis, A. E., Work, M., Barker, P. B., Jacobs, M. A., Breese, E. L., & Maurer, K. (2004). Re-examining the brain regions crucial for orchestrating speech articulation. *Brain*, 127, 1479–1487.

Jakobson, R. (1964). Toward a linguistic typology of aphasic impairments. In A. V. S. DeReuck & M. O'Connor (Eds.), *Disorders of language*. New York: Little & Brown.

Jakobson, R., & Halle, M. (1956). *Two aspects of language and two types of aphasic disturbances*. New York: Mouton.

Jonides, J., Smith, E. E., Koeppe, R. A., Awh, E., Minoshima, S., & Mintun, M. A. (1993). Spatial working memory in humans as revealed by PET. *Nature*, 363, 623–625.

Kandel, E. R., Schwartz, J. H., & Jessell, T. M. (1995). *Essentials of neural science and behavior*. Norwalk, CT: Appleton & Lange.

Kertesz, A. (1979). *Aphasia and associated disorders*. New York: Grune & Stratton.

Kertesz, A. (1982). *The Western Aphasia Battery*. New York: Grune & Stratton.

Kertesz, A. (1985). Aphasia. In J. A. M. Frederiks (Ed.), *Handbook of clinical neurology*, vol 45: Clinical neuropsychology. Amsterdam: Elsevier.

Kertesz, A. (2010). Ardila's attempt to alter aphasiology. *Aphasiology.* 24 (3), 404-407.

Kleist, K. (1934). *Gehirnpathologie*. Leipzig: Barth.

Kohn, S. (Ed.). (1992). *Conduction aphasia*. Mahwah, NJ: Lawrence Erlbaum Associates Inc.

Lebrun, Y. (1987). Anosognosia in aphasia. *Cortex*, 23, 251–263.

Lecours, A. R., Lhermitte, F., & Bryans, B. (1983). *Aphasiology*. London: Baillere-Tindall.

Lecours, A. R., Osborn, E., Travies, L., Rouillon, F., & Lavalle-Huyng, G. (1981). Jargons. In J. Brown (Ed.), *Jargonaphasia* (pp. 9–38). New York: Academic Press.

Lee, A., Kannan, V., & Hillis, A. E. (2006). The contribution of neuroimaging to the study of language and aphasia. *Neuropsychology Review*, 16, 171–183.

Lichtheim, L. (1885). On aphasia. *Brain*, 7, 433–484.

Luria, A. R. (1966). *Human brain and psychological processes.* New York: Harper & Row.

Luria, A. R. (1970). *Traumatic aphasia: Its syndromes, psychology, and treatment.* New York: Mouton.

Luria, A. R. (1974). *The working brain.* New York: Basic Books.

Luria, A. R. (1976). *Basic problems of neurolinguistics.* New York: Mouton.

Luria, A. R. (1980). *Higher cortical functions in man* (2nd ed.). New York: Basic Books.

Marshall, J. (2010). Classification of aphasia: Are there benefits for practice? *Aphasiology.* 24 (3), 408-412

Mellet, E., Tzourio, N., Crivello, F., Joliot, M., Denis, M., & Mazoyer, B. (1996). Functional anatomy of spatial mental imagery generated from verbal instructions. *Journal of Neuroscience,* 16, 6504–6512.

Meinzer,M., Harnish, S., Conway ,T., & Crosson, B. (2011). Recent developments in functional and structural imaging of aphasia recovery after stroke. *Aphasiology*, 25(3):271-290.

Paulesu, E., Frith, C. D., & Frackowiak, R. S. (1993). The neural correlates of the verbal component of working memory. *Nature,* 362, 342–345.

Penfield, W., & Welch, K. (1951). The supplementary motor area of the cerebral cortex: A clinical and experimental study. *AMA Archives of Neurology and Psychiatry*, 66, 289–317.

Pick, A. (1931). *Aphasia.* New York: Charles C. Thomas.

Rizzolatti, G., & Arbib, M. A. (1998). Language within our grasp. *Trends in Neurosciences,* 21, 188–194.

Robson, H., Keidel, J.L., Ralph, M.A. & Sage, K. (2012). Revealing and quantifying the impaired phonological analysis underpinning impaired comprehension in Wernicke's aphasia. Neuropsychologia, ;50(2):276-88.

Robson, H., Sage, K., & Ralph, M.A (2012). Wernicke's aphasia reflects a combination of acoustic-phonological and semantic control deficits: a case-series comparison of Wernicke's aphasia, semantic dementia and semantic aphasia. *Neuropsychologia,* 50(2):266-75.

Rubens, A. B. (1975). Aphasia with infarction in the territory of the anterior cerebral artery. *Cortex,* 11, 239–250.

Rubens, A. B. (1976). Transcortical motor aphasia. In H. Whitaker & H. A. Whitaker (Eds.), *Studies in neurolinguistics,* vol 1. New York: Academic Press.

Schuell, H. (1973). *Differential diagnosis of aphasia with the Minnesota Test.* Minneapolis, MN: University of Minnesota Press.

Simon, S. R., Meunier, M., Piettre, L., Berardi, A. M., Segebarth, C. M., & Boussaoud, D. (2002). Spatial attention and memory versus motor preparation: Premotor cortex involvement as revealed by fMRI. *Journal of Neurophysiology,* 88, 2047–2057.

Small, S. L., & Burton, M. W. (2002). Functional magnetic resonance imaging studies of language. *Current Neurology and Neuroscience Reports,* 2, 505–510.

Song, X., Dornbos, D., La,i Z., Zhang, Y., Li, T., Chen, H., Yang, Z. (2011). Diffusion tensor imaging and diffusion tensor imaging-fibre tractograph depict the mechanisms of Broca-like and Wernicke-like conduction aphasia. *Neurology Research,* 33, 529-35.

Taylor-Sarno, M. (1998). *Acquired aphasia.* New York: Academic Press.

Tesak, J., & Code, C. (2008). *Milestones in the history of aphasia: Theories and protagonists.* London: Psychology Press.

Ullman, M. T. (2004). Contributions of memory circuits to language: The declarative/ procedural model. *Cognition,* 92, 231–270.

Warabi, Y., Bandoh, M., Kurisaki, H., Nishio, S., & Hayashi, H. (2006). [Transcortical sensory aphasia due to extensive infarction of left cerebral hemisphere]. *Rinsho Shinkeigaku,* 46, 317–321.

Wernicke, C. (1874). *Der Aphasiche Symptomencomplex.* Breslau: Cohn & Weigert.

Wilson, S. A. K. (1926). *Aphasia.* London: Kegan Paul.

Yamada, K., Nagakane, Y., Mizuno, T., Hosomi, A., Nakagawa, M., & Nishimura, T. (2007). MR tractography depicting damage to the arcuate fasciculus in a patient with conduction aphasia. *Neurology,* 68, 789–790.

Zahn, R., Huber, W., Drews, E., Erberich, S., Krings, T., & Willmes, K. et al. (2000). Hemispheric lateralization at different levels of human auditory word processing: A functional magnetic resonance imaging study. *Neuroscience Letters,* 287, 195–198.

Index

beneficial effect, 74, 80
benefits, 79, 92, 103, 133
blood, 77, 87
blood flow, 87
blood pressure, 77
body schema, 106
brain damage, 35, 50, 87
breakdown, 35, 104

C

calcium, 80
candidates, 84
capsule, 60
carbon, 48
carbon monoxide, 48
cardiomyopathy, 46, 66
caregivers, vii, x, 1, 3, 14, 26, 33, 39, 52, 55, 62, 92, 103
caregiving, 3, 36
case study, 65, 130
causation, 47
CBD, 53
cell death, 62
central nervous system, ix, 69
cerebral arteries, 126
cerebral cortex, 133
cerebral edema, 50
cerebral function, 93
cerebral hemisphere, 42, 95, 134
cerebrovascular disease, 86
chaos, 29
Chicago, 38
children, 5, 27, 30
cholinesterase, 72, 80
cholinesterase inhibitors, 80
classification, vii, x, 43, 102, 115, 116, 117, 128
clinical application, 87
clinical disorders, 124
clinical examination, 110
clinical syndrome, 52, 118, 119
CNS, viii, 41, 87, 88, 96
coffee, 31
cognition, 56, 79, 116, 124

cognitive ability, 22, 124
cognitive impairment, 52, 60, 109
cognitive tasks, 127
collaboration, 92
communication, ix, 3, 5, 7, 8, 11, 12, 13, 17, 18, 19, 20, 21, 22, 24, 26, 28, 29, 30, 33, 34, 35, 36, 43, 70, 72, 74, 81, 92, 102, 103, 104
communication skills, 11, 33
community, viii, 2, 3, 5, 22, 24, 25, 26, 30, 31, 32, 34, 35, 37, 61
community service, viii, 2, 3, 5, 22, 25, 26, 30, 31, 32, 35, 37
compensation, 101
complement, 21, 36
complexity, 6, 27
compliance, 50
complications, 106
comprehension, vii, viii, 42, 43, 45, 46, 47, 48, 49, 51, 53, 64, 74, 79, 100, 119, 122, 123, 125, 133
computer, ix, 70, 71, 73, 75, 83, 85, 86, 87, 88, 90
computer-assisted therapy (CAT), ix, 70, 73, 83
conduction, x, 47, 58, 59, 115, 121, 122, 123, 128, 129, 130, 131, 134
confrontation, 20
connectivity, 71
consciousness, 11, 15, 28, 93
constraint-induced aphasia therapy (CIAT), ix, 70, 73, 74
consulting, 25
contiguity, 118, 120
control group, 74, 103, 104
controlled studies, 77, 104
controlled trials, 92, 104
controversial, ix, 77, 92
convention, 16
conversations, 22
cooperation, 24, 34, 105
coordination, x, 92, 105
correlation(s), viii, 42, 43, 52, 57, 59, 60, 66, 72, 95, 100, 109

infarction, 45, 59, 60, 76, 89, 102, 106, 110, 134
inferiority, vii, 1, 16, 23, 24, 34
inhibition, 82
inhibitor, 77
initiation, 102, 103
injury(s), viii, 26, 27, 28, 30, 35, 69, 71, 94, 100, 129
insecurity, 17
integrity, 24, 36
intelligence, 28
intentionality, 15, 16
intercourse, 5
interference, ix, 70
interpersonal communication, 36
interpersonal relations, 2, 13, 17, 23, 27, 28, 34, 52
interpersonal relationships, 52
intervention, ix, 70, 72, 81, 106
intonation, 83, 90, 103, 112
intracerebral hemorrhage, 93, 97
intracranial aneurysm, 108
inventiveness, 28
irritability, 55
ischemia, 86
islands, 42
isolation, 3, 8, 18, 19, 36, 47, 48, 130
issues, viii, 2, 4, 24, 32, 34, 35, 42, 82, 87

J

Japan, 110

L

language impairment, vii, 20, 46, 52, 53, 63, 93, 94, 95, 99, 102, 111, 118, 125, 126
language processing, 95, 116
language skills, 72
languages, 87
larynx, 95
latency, 78
Latin America, 116

lead, ix, 2, 29, 53, 54, 72, 92
learning, ix, 70, 71, 72, 75, 76, 77, 80, 81, 84, 85, 87, 89, 90
learning process, 73
left hemisphere, viii, 42, 71, 82, 94, 100, 101, 121, 125, 126
lesions, 42, 44, 45, 46, 47, 49, 50, 60, 100, 101, 125, 126
level of education, 101
lexical processing, 60
life expectancy, 52
light, 13, 19, 28
localization, 100
loneliness, 3, 13, 16, 17, 23, 24, 28, 33, 36
love, 25, 27, 28, 33

M

magnetic field, 82
magnetic resonance, 100, 134
magnetic resonance imaging, 100, 134
magnetoencephalography, 131
majority, viii, 42, 52, 101
man, 7, 8, 11, 12, 25, 28, 38, 58, 102, 131, 133
management, vii, viii, ix, 2, 36, 43, 56, 92, 94
manipulation, 51
mapping, 60, 112, 130
Martin Heidegger, 35
Maryland, 66, 108
mass, 50
matter, 9, 10, 36, 71, 73, 106, 112, 116
MB, 109
medical, 23, 55, 103, 105
melody, 44
memory, 52, 55, 56, 76, 77, 79, 80, 86, 87, 108, 119, 127, 134
memory loss, 55
mental image, 127, 133
mental imagery, 127, 133
mental processes, 8
Merleau-Ponty, 15, 32, 33, 38
messages, 11, 14, 23
meta analysis, 73

Q

R

U

V

W

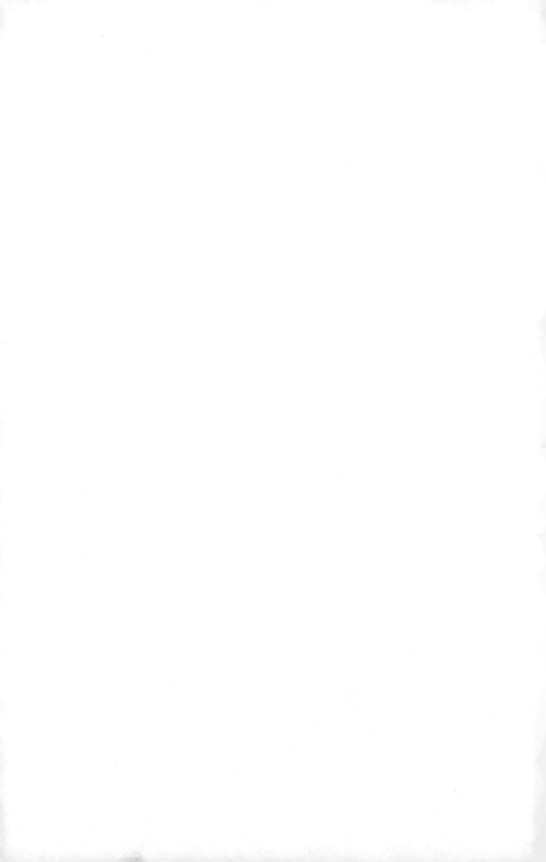

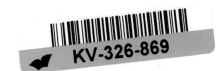
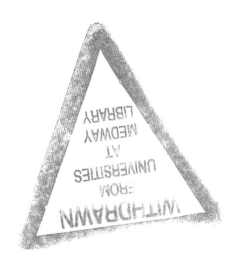

AGENDAS FOR SUSTAINABILITY

Does anyone really know how to save the Earth?

Despite the avalanche of agendas for sustainable development set off by the Earth Summit in Rio, the Earth now seems to be in worse rather than better shape. No government, NGO, business or other major player has been able to implement all the recommendations in even one of the agendas set.

Yet the very experience of setting the agendas may be their greatest legacy, indicating that although there is common ground among groups, there are also real differences in belief systems that motivate people to work for sustainable development. This book argues that the courage to expose these differences and the creativity to resolve them are central to the successful revitalization of the sustainable development movement.

Agendas for Sustainability looks at the value of setting agendas as a mechanism for social change. It identifies similarities and differences among eleven sustainable development agendas including *Agenda 21*, the *NGO Alternative Treaties*, and the IUCN/UNEP/WWF publication *Caring for the Earth*. Points of divergence and areas of common ground are investigated in over thirty environment- and development-related topics, including biodiversity, consumption patterns, urbanization, population, education and water resources. Reporting on the fate of these agendas in the aftermath of Rio, this book uncovers the principal obstacles to change and examines why so little progress has been achieved.

Mary MacDonald is Director of Policy and Research at the Earth Council and an Affiliated Scientist of the Stockholm Environment Institute.

ROUTLEDGE/SEI GLOBAL ENVIRONMENT AND
DEVELOPMENT SERIES
Series Editor: Arno Rosemarin

SOCIETIES AND NATURE IN THE SAHEL
Claude Raynaut, Emmanuel Gregoire, Pierre Janin, Jean Koechlin and
Philippe Lavigne Delville

AGENDAS FOR SUSTAINABILITY: ENVIRONMENT AND
DEVELOPMENT INTO THE TWENTY-FIRST CENTURY
Mary MacDonald

AGENDAS FOR SUSTAINABILITY

Environment and development into the
twenty-first century

Mary ⌊MacDonald

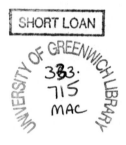

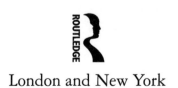

London and New York

First published 1998
by Routledge
11 New Fetter Lane, London EC4P 4EE

Simultaneously published in the USA and Canada
by Routledge
29 West 35th Street, New York, NY 10001

Typeset in Garamond by
M Rules
Printed and bound in Great Britain by
Biddles Ltd, Guildford and King's Lynn

British Library Cataloguing in Publication Data
A catalogue record for this book is available from the British Library

Library of Congress Cataloging in Publication Data
MacDonald, Mary, 1961–
Agendas for sustainability: environment and development into
the 21st century / Mary MacDonald
p. cm.
Includes bibliographical references and index.
1. Environmental policy. 2. Sustainable development. I. Title.
GE170.M33 1998
363.7–dc21 97-35355
CIP

ISBN 0 415 15491 X

This is a moment of hope in history. Why doesn't anybody say so?
P.J. O'Rourke, *All the Trouble in the World*, 1994

CONTENTS

CONTENTS

TABLES

FOREWORD

by Maurice Strong
Chairman of the Earth Council

The United Nations Conference on Environment and Development held in Rio de Janeiro in June 1992, twenty years after the Stockholm Conference on the Human Environment, focused attention on the multifaceted and international nature of many environment and development issues. At UNCED, in particular, the local national and global aspects of environment- and development-related problems were brought to the fore. Against the backdrop of a growing awareness of the negative impacts of some of the current approaches to development, 177 governments approved an agreement, known as Agenda 21, outlining a programme for working towards a 'global partnership for sustainable development'.

But governments are not the only ones dedicated to building a more sustainable future. Even before the Stockholm Conference in 1972 many individuals were organizing around environment and development issues that were either affecting them directly in their everyday lives or for which they felt a moral responsibility to take action. People from different backgrounds have different ways of understanding and experiencing these issues. Evidence of this can be found among the many agendas for environment and development that were proposed around the time of the negotiations for *Agenda 21* and contributed to it.

It is heartening to see the level of agreement among the different groups who proposed the agendas considered in this study. And it is an optimistic sign that so many people were, and remain, interested enough to think seriously about the issues and propose workable solutions. The agendas discussed here are just a sampling of the many proposals for a more sustainable future. But they do give an indication of a growing consensus for change. *Agenda 21*, as the confirmed agenda adopted by governments, is the primary reference point.

As the recent United Nations General Assembly Special Session on progress since the Earth Summit indicated, a great deal remains to be done towards implementing sustainability. As we work to gain a better understanding of just what achieving this goal will require we can look to studies such as *Shared Hope* to see how many insightful and learned suggestions have already been made – and to remind ourselves that, while our own situation may be unique in many ways, we are not alone in our desire to create a more secure and equitable world for future generations.

ACKNOWLEDGEMENTS

This book would not have been possible without generous gifts of time, skill and, of course, funding from many sources. I would like to thank the Stockholm Environment Institute, Sweden and the Earth Council, Costa Rica for providing financial and institutional support for the research undertaken here. Alicia Barcéna, former Executive Director of the Earth Council and Mike Chadwick, former Director of the Stockholm Environment Institute, both offered much inspiration and encouragement during the important start-up phase of the project, for which I am grateful.

Earlier drafts of the manuscript benefited from interviews with and comments from a great number of people. In particular, I would like to thank Patricia Araneta, Alicia Barcéna, Nicola Brookes, Sarah Burns, Mike Chadwick, Hugh Faulkner, Elizabeth Garfunkel, Alvin Manitopyes, Julia Marton-LeFevre, Francisco Mata, Jeff McNeeley, Peter Padbury, Nic Robins, Michael Small and the two anonymous reviewers appointed by the publishers, Routledge.

The enthusiasm of Nick Sonntag, the current Executive Director of the Stockholm Environment Institute, was instrumental in propelling me to update and complete the work. I am also thankful for the unflagging help I have received from Arno Rosemarin, Director of Communications at SEI. Valerie Rose and Kate Chenevix Trench at Routledge deserve recognition for their patience and commitment to the project as does Erik Willis for his creative work on the graphics for the book.

My colleagues at the Stockholm Environment Institute at York participated in many hours of thoughtful discussion on various aspects of the book. For their intellectual input and, above all, their friendship I would like to thank Johan Kuylenstierna, Annie Christie, Peter Bailey, Clair Gough, Steve Cinderby, 'H' Cambridge, Harry Vallack, and Erik Willis.

Finally, it was my good fortune to work with two people who went way beyond the call of duty in their contributions to the project. I am very thankful for the dedication and tireless attention to detail shown by my dear friend Isobel Devane who so good-naturedly produced the manuscript, several times over. I am also grateful to the talented and, at times necessarily, ruthless John

Chenery whose creative suggestions helped me rework a much larger monograph into a more reasonable format and whose clear and careful editing transformed the manuscript from a rather mundane report to a more lively offering.

ABBREVIATIONS AND ACRONYMS

ADEL	Agencies of Local Economic Development
AIDS	acquired immune deficiency syndrome
AIESEC	*Association Internationale des Etudiants en Science Economique*
ASCEND 21	An Agenda of Science for Environment and Development into the Twenty-first Century
BCSD	Business Council for Sustainable Development
CBD	Convention on Biological Diversity
CFC	chlorofluorohydrocarbon
CO_2	carbon dioxide
COWAN	Country Women Association of Nigeria
CSD	Commission on Sustainable Development
ELCI	Environmental Liaison Centre International
ESW	Earth Summit Watch
FAO	Food and Agriculture Organization
GATT	General Agreement on Tariffs and Trade
GEF	Global Environment Facility
GIS	Geographical Information Systems
GSS	Global Seminar Series (AIESEC)
GTOS	Global Terrestrial Observing System
HIV	human immunodeficiency virus
IAEA	International Atomic Energy Agency
IAWQ	International Association on Water Quality
ICLEI	International Council for Local Environment Initiatives
ICPD	International Conference on Population and Development
ICSU	International Council of Scientific Unions
IGBP	International Geosphere-Biosphere Programme
IGOs	Intergovernmental Organizations
IHDP	International Human Dimensions of Global Change Programme
IIED	International Institute for Environment and Development
ILO	International Labour Organization
IMF	International Monetary Fund

IPF	Intergovernmental panel on forests
IPR	intellectual property rights
ISRIC	International Soil Reference and Information Centre
ISSC	International Social Science Council
IUCN	The World Conservation Union (formerly International Union for the Conservation of Nature and Natural Resources)
LCA	life-cycle analysis
MSC	Marine Stewardship Council
MSWICI	Morgan Stanley World International Capital Index
NAFTA	North American Free Trade Agreement
NGOs	non-governmental organizations
ODA	Official Development Assistance
OECD	Organization for Economic Co-operation and Development
POs	people's organizations
PREPCOM	Preparatory Committee Meeting for UNCED
SCOPE	Scientific Committee on Problems of the Environment
SEI	Stockholm Environment Institute
TEMS	Terrestrial Ecosystem Monitoring Sites Database
TNCs	Transnational Corporations
TWAS	Third World Academy of Sciences
UN	United Nations
UNCED	United Nations Conference on Environment and Development
UNCTAD	United Nations Conference on Trade and Development
UNDP	United Nations Development Programme
UNEP	United Nations Environment Programme
UNESCO	United Nations Educational, Scientific and Cultural Organization
UNGASS	United Nations General Assembly Special Session
USAID	United States Agency for International Development
WBCSD	World Business Council for Sustainable Development
WCRP	World Climate Research Programme
WEDO	Women's Environment and Development Organization
WHO	World Health Organization
WRI	World Resources Institute
WTO	World Trade Organization
WWF	World Wide Fund for Nature (also called World Wildlife Fund)

1

A BIG BUILD-UP

Gun-toting soldiers perched atop buildings and hillsides surrounded by sand-bags and radar aerials while down at ground level a Zen master painted Chinese characters defining the personality traits of passers-by. This milling throng included celebrities like Jane Fonda, Pelé, Jacques Cousteau and Shirley MacLaine. Inside there was a VIP area called the 'golden corridor'. Outside, the poor and homeless had already been rounded up and shipped across the bay, out of sight and, for two weeks at least, out of mind.

So what was all the fuss about? For months the international media had been enchanted by this thing called the United Nations Conference on Environment and Development. The week before it began, it had filled more than fifteen pages in *Time* and *Newsweek*. During the event, there were daily front-page reports in every major newspaper in the world and footage on every television newscast.

This was the Earth Summit. It was held in June 1992 in Rio de Janeiro, where more than 100 heads of state and delegations from over 170 countries had come to put the finishing touches on what was being billed as an agenda for the twenty-first century. Along with national delegations and accredited media, more than 30,000 people with no official status at the UN Conference on Environment and Development also descended upon Rio. Many of them were involved in their own negotiations of 'alternative treaties'.

The watching world, subjected nightly to images of rainforests falling and wildlife disappearing, could have been forgiven for thinking that the conference was only about the environment. But this was to be a very different animal. The Earth Summit was designed to combine wise management and conservation of the natural environment with economic equity and access to basic needs for all people. And somehow it had to find a way to mesh these seemingly competing goals in a manner that would allow them to be pursued in perpetuity.

Some history

The 1962 publication of Rachel Carson's *Silent Spring*,[1] in which she made a powerful argument for the link between pesticide use, widespread pollution

1

and the resultant devastating effects on the health of humans and other animals and plants, is often cited as the moment the environmental movement began to take shape. From that point onward there has been a growing awareness of the need to balance human needs with the well-being of the natural world.

By the end of the 1960s the United Nations was discussing environmental issues[2] and in 1972 the United Nations Conference on the Human Environment was held in Stockholm. This meeting highlighted the different approaches of developed and developing countries to environment and development, many of which continue to this day.[3] The Stockholm Conference is credited with the emergence of environmental policies and accompanying institutional support including environment and natural resource ministries in many countries. The United Nations Environment Programme was also created in its aftermath.

The Stockholm Conference resulted in two documents – the *Stockholm Declaration on Human Environment* and the *Action Plan for the Human Environment* – which were among the earliest government-sanctioned attempts to set an agenda for global action in response to environment and development problems. Yet they did not contain a clear recognition of the universal nature of environment and development issues. Over the next twenty years it would become startlingly obvious that many activities undertaken in one part of the globe could have profound consequences in another part of the world or could damage common resources such as the atmosphere or the oceans.

'Globalization' is the term often used to describe the rapid movement towards an integrated global market.[4] But economic activity is not the only global phenomenon to be recognized in recent years. The depletion of the ozone layer was the first global environmental issue for which an international accord was struck. In the *Montreal Protocol on Substances that Deplete the Ozone Layer* (1987; revised 1990) processes and products involving chlorofluorohydrocarbons and related substances are controlled and restricted by nations according to an agreed schedule. During the mid-1980s more and more scientists and then governments expressed concern about the build-up of carbon dioxide in the atmosphere and its potential to change the climate. The loss of genetic diversity which accompanied the clearing of large tracts of land for agriculture and other types of development around the globe was also being recognized.

The publication of *Our Common Future*, the report of the World Commission on Environment and Development[5] (known as the Brundtland Commission after its chair, Gro Harlem Brundtland), provided another boost to international interest in sustainable development. *Our Common Future* was released in 1987 after a series of consultations in many countries featuring the input of people from different backgrounds including government, environmental and development NGOs, business, education, indigenous peoples' groups and academia. The mandate of the World Commission on Environment and Development was to formulate 'a global agenda for change'. The Commission put forward a working definition of sustainable development, the value of which is still debated. The report stated that,

> In essence, sustainable development is a process of change in which the exploitation of resources, the direction of investments, the orientation of technological development and institutional change are all in harmony and enhance both current and future potential to meet human needs and aspirations.

By the twentieth anniversary of the Stockholm Conference, marked by the United Nations Conference on Environment and Development, it was accepted that there were a number of problems which could only be labelled as global and to which the most appropriate response was a global one. The Earth Summit resulted in five major documents, including a declaration, *The Rio Declaration on Environment and Development*, two conventions – *The Convention on Biological Diversity* and *The United Nations Framework Convention on Climate Change* – a statement, *Statement of Principles on Forests*, and a broad, detailed, 400-page plan of action known as *Agenda 21*.[6]

The Earth Summit was a milestone in inducing governments to address the relationships between environment and development rather than view them as separate issues. It was also a time of great optimism. Ambassador Razali Ismail of Malaysia, an outspoken representative for developing countries at Rio and President of the UN General Assembly in 1997, recalls: 'I recognize 1992 as the time when all of us hit the zenith of commitment on environment and development'.[7]

At the Earth Summit, *Agenda 21* was hailed as the blueprint for a better world. More than 170 governments committed themselves to it, although their signature was not binding and the plan of action did not require ratification. Five years later the Statement of Commitment from Earth Summit +5, a United Nations General Assembly Special Session on progress since the Earth Summit, pronounced:

> We acknowledge that a number of positive results have been achieved, but we are deeply concerned that the overall trends for sustainable development are worse today than they were in 1992. We emphasize that the implementation of *Agenda 21* in a comprehensive manner remains vitally important and is more urgent now than ever.[8]

Emergence of agendas

By the time early drafts of *Agenda 21* started circulating to begin government negotiations, a number of other agendas were being brought forward by global networks of NGOs, grassroots organizations, the science and academic communities, the private sector and indigenous peoples. The purpose of this book

3

is to assess the value of agenda-setting as a means for moving to a more sustainable future. The agendas used for this investigation are:

- *Agenda 21*
- *The NGO Alternative Treaties*[9]
- *Agenda Ya Wananchi: Citizens' Action Plan for the 1990s*[10]
- *Agenda of Science for Environment and Development into the Twenty-first Century*[11]
- *Caring for the Earth: A Strategy for Sustainable Living*[12]
- *Women's Action Agenda 21*[13]
- *The Global Assembly of Women and the Environment*[14]
- *Youth '92: The World Youth Preparatory Forum for UNCED*[15]
- *Youth Action Guide on Sustainable Development*[16]
- *Voice of the Eagle: The Final Warning Message of the Indigenous People of Mother Earth*[17]
- *Changing Course: A Global Business Perspective on Development and Environment*[18]

All these agendas came into being in the two years before UNCED. Several of them supported lobbying efforts during the UNCED process, particularly with respect to the government agreement, *Agenda 21*. All stressed the need to question prevailing priorities and actions in the many areas relating to environment and development.

Taken together, the eleven agendas listed above amount to around 1,500 pages of statements, goals and recommended actions for achieving sustainable development (and they are not the only agendas that came forward at the time of UNCED). Why did so many people put their time and talents into drafting agendas for environment and development? Perhaps the success of the *Montreal Protocol on Ozone* made it appear that the political climate was ripe to take action on the underlying causes of environmental destruction and social deprivation. *The Montreal Protocol* had given governments experience in talking about and negotiating on a complex issue which had economic, social and ecological dimensions.

The general public, too, had become more sensitive than ever before to the threats posed by unchecked industrial activity in many parts of the globe. In the early 1980s it was recognized that acid rain was crossing national borders in North America and northern Europe and killing lakes in countries where it was not being produced. People already knew about the depletion of the ozone layer and, by the early 1990s, they were also hearing a great deal about carbon dioxide emissions and their link with climate change.

More than ever before, people were asking questions about the reasons for these problems and the answers were seldom straightforward. It seemed impossible to talk about cutting carbon dioxide emissions, for example, without addressing economic losses or social impacts such as the loss of jobs.

4

Within this context, many people saw the United Nations Conference on Environment and Development as an opportunity to push their ideas for change. Organized groups, particularly those familiar with political lobbying, set about putting their suggestions into formal documents. And so many agendas came into being, some quite similar, others completely different but all with two things in common. They all asked, and in many cases, demanded, a change. They all shared hope.

2

THE AGENDA-SETTING PROCESS

With the exception of government delegations, most of the agendas were prepared by a self-selected group – that is, individuals who were motivated to participate in working for change rather than elected to represent a certain constituency. These people felt confident that they could speak in a representative fashion for the group with which they were most strongly affiliated. Many of the documents underwent a relatively lengthy drafting process which included broad consultation within a given sector.

Agenda 21

Prior to UNCED, four Preparatory Committee (PREPCOM) meetings were held involving the UNCED Secretariat, interested government delegations and observers. *Agenda 21* was first put forward as a discussion document by the UNCED Secretariat between the second and third PREPCOM. The initial document was much shorter in length and narrower in scope than the final version. All the chapters of *Agenda 21* were, in theory, reviewed by government delegations to UNCED and were modified to varying degrees until the final text was agreed upon in Rio by 177 governments.

Because of the large numbers of people involved in negotiating *Agenda 21* it is not clear precisely whose ideas the documents represent. The first draft of *Agenda 21* put forward by the UNCED Secretariat benefited from input from meetings of the Secretariat staff with groups of experts from both non-governmental and intergovernmental organizations from all parts of the globe on a variety of environment and development issues. The Brundtland Commission Report, *Our Common Future* (1987), was also available to draw upon for the first draft.

As the Agenda took shape, government delegations including diplomats and, as resources allowed, national experts from relevant disciplines, became the primary force for revising chapters, including adding and removing ideas and emphasis, in conjunction with an active and hard-working secretariat. Senior government officials who participated in UNCED were primarily part of ministries or institutes concerned with the regulation of national resources such as water, minerals or forests as well as public works, transport, tourism and housing, rather than the more powerful decision-making portfolios of finance or trade and industry.

UNCED documents were first presented in English and, although translations were eventually prepared in many languages, the final documents may, in some way, reflect that some inputs were not possible due to a lack of timely translations.

NGO Alternative Treaties

The 'Alternative Treaty Making Process' was begun in Paris in 1991 at the time of the third PREPCOM by NGO groups who felt that *Agenda 21* would not fill 'the growing gap between the interest of states and politicians and the interest of communities and civil society institutions'.[19] The work was co-ordinated by the International NGO Forum, a group of fewer than twenty intellectually endowed activists with a great deal of experience in their own countries as well as internationally. The Treaties were signed by more than 3,000 NGOs and people's organizations (POs).

Guidelines prepared for the Alternative Treaty Making Process emphasize that any treaty must present views from both the South and the North and include a co-ordinator from each of these regions. Most of the treaty negotiation was completed in four days. Negotiations took place at the Global Forum attended by 30,000 people and held concurrently with UNCED. The emphasis was on the formation of principles and commitments, and it was made clear that signatories were not necessarily bound by all points contained in a treaty. Since much of the exercise took place in Brazil there was a high proportion of treaty negotiators from that country but there was also a broad representation of NGOs and POs from all parts of the globe. The *NGO Alternative Treaties* did not result from a full process that paralleled exactly the process of *Agenda 21*. Far fewer people were involved in developing the treaties and, in many cases, the treaties were the work of a handful of individuals with a special interest in the treaty topic. The *NGO Alternative Treaties* were also initially produced only in English. Translations were subsequently available in Spanish, French and Portuguese.

Agenda Ya Wananchi

Agenda Ya Wananchi: Citizens' Action Plan for the 1990s is the published outcome of a meeting of citizens' movements called the Roots of the Future which was held in Paris in December 1991. The conference was organized to support NGO activity at the Earth Summit. Financial support for the document came from the Ford Foundation, USAID, UNDP, UNEP and the governments of France, the Netherlands, Sweden, Norway and Finland.

The Agenda itself was based on the *Compendium of Citizens' Movements*

Responses to Environment and Development Challenges, a report compiled following meetings with hundreds of local, regional, national and international citizens' groups and three round-table discussions held in mid-1991. Those attending the Roots of the Future, which included more than 1,200 people from more than 150 nations, were given the draft version of *Agenda Ya Wananchi*, which was discussed and modified during the conference proceedings. The published agenda was co-ordinated by the Environment and Development Resource Centre, Belgium, and synthesized and revised by nine individuals from citizen's groups operating in different parts of the globe (India (two), Poland, Norway, Argentina, USA (two), Kenya, the Netherlands). *Agenda Ya Wananchi* was originally produced in English, Spanish and French and later translated into Portuguese and Arabic.

Agenda of Science for Environment and Development into the Twenty-first Century (ASCEND 21)

ASCEND 21 is the output from a conference organized by the International Council of Scientific Unions (ICSU), Stockholm Environment Institute (SEI) and others, held in Vienna in November 1991. ICSU was asked in September 1990, by the Secretary-General of UNCED, to act as 'principal scientific adviser in the preparation of Rio UNCED'. Following this request, ICSU made a substantial contribution to the UNCED Working Group on Science for Sustainable Development and ICSU scientists also participated in a number of other UNCED working groups preparing *Agenda 21* chapters. ICSU actively encouraged scientists in all parts of the globe to become involved in their national contributions to UNCED. As well, ICSU decided to organize a conference of the scientific community (to include national, social, engineering and health scientists) to apply current levels of knowledge and judgement towards understanding 'the all important linkages between environment and development'.

More than 250 scientists from nearly seventy countries participated in *ASCEND 21*. Those who attended the *ASCEND 21* conference were selected by the ICSU advisory committee. Names were put forward for involvement in the proceedings by the sponsoring organizations (Third World Academy of Sciences, European Science Foundation, International Institute for Applied Systems Analysis, International Social Science Council, Norwegian Council for Science and Humanities, Norwegian Academy of Science and Letters, Stockholm Environment Institute) and by UN agencies. The results of *ASCEND 21* are based on sixteen papers prepared by teams of two or three authors, modified and supplemented by discussions at a meeting of authors held four months prior to the conference and the working group sessions held at ASCEND in November. Most of the sixteen chapters in *ASCEND 21* are co-authored by a scientist from a developing country and one scientist from a developed country. *ASCEND 21* is available only in English.

8

Caring for the Earth: A Strategy for Sustainable Living

Ten years ago IUCN, UNEP and WWF published a World Conservation Strategy emphasizing the belief that 'conservation is not the opposite of development'[20] and introducing the term 'sustainable development' into general use.[21] *Caring for the Earth*, which required two years of preparation, built on and revised some of the main points contained in the World Conservation Strategy as well as offering new ideas. Staff members from the three sponsoring organizations assisted in preparing the two draft versions of the strategy, with IUCN taking principal responsibility for the preparation of the text.

The primary force behind *Caring for the Earth: A Strategy for Sustainable Living* appears to be IUCN, including input from its many governmental and non-governmental members. UNEP and WWF were also key participants in preparation of the strategy. The strategy was the result of specialist workshops and consultations with over a dozen organizations including UN agencies such as the FAO, Habitat, international and regional banks such as the Asian Development Bank and the World Bank, and environmental organizations such as WRI and IIED. The names of approximately 900 individuals who provided comments on draft versions of the strategy are listed at the end of the document but there is no indication of the affiliation of these commentators. *Caring for the Earth* is available in English, French and Spanish.

Women's Action Agenda 21

The *Women's Action Agenda 21* was part of the outcome of the World Women's Congress for a Healthy Planet which took place in November 1991 in Miami. The conference was organized by the Women's Environment and Development Organization (WEDO) under the guidance of the Women's International Policy Action Committee, which was made up of fifty-four women from thirty-one countries. WEDO is a programme of the Women's Foreign Policy Council/Women USA Fund Inc., a non-profit organization which began in New York in 1980. The document was 'specifically designed to promote women's active and equal participation for the June 1992 United Nations Conference on Environment and Development (UNCED) in Brazil, and in implementing its expected plan of action, *Agenda 21*'.

Participants of the Women's World Congress for a Healthy Planet including 1,500 women from eighty-three countries received a draft version of the *Women's Action Agenda 21* upon arrival. This draft was prepared in consultation with groups, lawyers and activists with a special interest in women, environment and development. The final version of the agenda built on this initial draft and included ideas from the many discussions and workshops held during the congress, although the editors included a note indicating that the agenda 'represented the essence' of discussion and that it 'does not necessarily represent

9

the views of each and every individual who participated'. All working documents and the final draft were available in English, French and Spanish.

Global Assembly of Women and the Environment

The report entitled *The Global Assembly of Women and the Environment: Partners in Life* is the outcome of four regional conferences held between February 1989 and March 1991 as part of the United Nations Environment Programme's response to the 1985 World Conference to Review and Appraise the Achievements of the United Nations Decade for Women. In addition, the Global Assembly, which was sponsored by the Senior Women's Advisory Group to the Executive Director of the United Nations Environment Programme, sought to 'demonstrate women's capacities in environmental management as they relate to global ecological issues, which include water, waste, energy and environmentally-friendly systems, products and technologies' by identifying and presenting 218 'grassroots success stories' from all parts of the globe. A final meeting took place in November 1991 in Miami.

The final report of the assembly includes success stories presented by women from five regions (Africa, Asia and the Pacific, Europe, Latin America and the Caribbean and North America) and recommendations and actions from a group called 'mentors' coming from the academic community, corporations, foundations, international agencies, national governments and NGOs. The final report also includes ideas from young women from around the globe, referred to in this document as 'new generation leaders'. Close to 500 people participated in the assembly.

Youth '92: the World Youth Preparatory Forum for UNCED

The *Youth '92* document is the result of a World Youth Preparatory Forum for UNCED, held in San José, Costa Rica, in March 1992. Preparation for this meeting included two years of national and regional youth events throughout the globe. Financial support for the project originated from the Canadian, Swedish and Danish governments, from the United Nations Environment Programme and small donations from participants and local supporters.

The conference participants included approximately 300 people between the ages of 15 and 30, 75 per cent of whom were from the South. Close to half of the attendees were women, and indigenous young people made up 10 per cent of those taking part. Those in attendance represented a wide range of religious, political, ethnic, cultural and geographical diversity, as well as including representatives from small local community groups and larger organizations. The organizers have called the World Youth Preparatory Forum 'one of the most representative youth activities of the decade'. During the conference the content of the document was finalized and consensus was reached in a variety of formal and less structured meetings. Final approval was given during plenary sessions. The preparatory documents and the statement and action plan were available in English, French and Spanish.

Youth Action Guide on Sustainable Development

The *Youth Action Guide on Sustainable Development* was produced following a World Theme Conference on Sustainable Development organized by the International Students' Organization, AIESEC (*Association Internationale des Etudiants en Science Economique*), in August 1990, in Tokyo. The conference followed over fifty seminars on sustainable development held in all parts of the globe. Together these were known as the AIESEC Global Seminar Series (GSS), and it was out of these meetings that the topics for the workshops at the World Theme Conference were developed. Shell International Petroleum Company was the major sponsor of the GSS and the printing of the *Youth Action Guide*. The World Theme Conference received sponsorship from over 100 government agencies, foundations, industrial associations, corporations and companies, the vast majority of which were Japanese.

Approximately 200 delegates from forty-five countries attended the conference, with roughly 25 per cent of the participants coming from developing countries. The majority of those who attended were economic and business students who had participated in the AIESEC GSS. Their 'limited knowledge of the issues' was supplemented by more than twenty speakers from business, industry, science and academia. During the workshops at the conference, discussion was focused on clarifying the problems associated with a particular issue, posing solutions and identifying activities that would support the solutions, with a special emphasis on actions that would be suitable for young people. The final guide was edited by two of the conference participants (one from the International Chamber of Commerce Office of Environment and Energy/International Bureau in Oslo, Norway; the other from McMaster University's Business Career Services in Hamilton, Canada). The *Youth Action Guide* is only available in English.

Voice of the Eagle

The publication known as *Voice of the Eagle: The Final Warning Message of the Indigenous People of Turtle Island Presented to the People of Mother Earth* (copyright Alvin Manitopyes and Dave Courchene, Jr) was commissioned by the International Indigenous Commission. It was sponsored by the Ira Hill Foundation and the Manitou Foundation and published by the Calgary Aboriginal Awareness Society. The Turtle Island referred to in the title is North America.

The work is a communication of spiritual beliefs and includes warnings and

11

advice about the health of the planet, referred to as Mother Earth. The two authors, members of the Plains Cree Nation and Anishnawbe Nation, acknowledge that they are only the carriers of the message and make no claim to be the originators. They are repeating the ideas of the ancestors and community elders who have a spiritual knowledge and understanding, through the Eagle Spirit which is known to be the Sacred Messenger of the Creator and 'symbolizes the power of the Creator's love'.

Changing Course

Changing Course: A Global Business Perspective on Development and Environment is a Business Council for Sustainable Development (BCSD) report on integrating environmental protection and economic growth. Stephan Schmidheiny is the principal author of *Changing Course* and chairman of a Swiss company called UNOTEC. In 1990 he was asked by Maurice Strong, Secretary-General of UNCED, to take on three tasks. These included:

- to serve as his principal adviser for business and industry;
- to present a global business perspective on sustainable development, and involve the international business community to stimulate the interest.

One of Schmidheiny's responses was to set up BSCD in mid-1990.

The World Business Council for Sustainable Development consists of forty-eight top executives of multinational corporations, 96 per cent of whom were men at the time *Changing Course* was put together. The Council organized over fifty different meetings (such as conferences, symposia, issue workshops) in twenty countries with representation from and participation of Africa, Asia and Latin America as well as Europe and North America. At the time, the council found it difficult to locate a developed 'business sector' in Eastern Europe, the former USSR and China, so those regions did not take part in council activities. Neither were small businesses or co-operatives represented.

There were three plenary sessions prior to the finalization of the report. At the first plenary a list of issues was agreed upon and task forces were given responsibility for reporting on certain topics. Consultants and writers outside the group were hired to produce draft chapters on a variety of topics. The editorial adviser was a senior staff member at the International Institute for Environment and Development (IIED).

The introduction to the book stresses that *Changing Course* 'is not a consensus document' but that the ideas and concepts presented were 'generally endorsed'. It was published, prior to the United Nations Conference on Environment and Development, in English, German, Spanish, Italian, Japanese and Portuguese and eventually published in a total of fifteen languages.

Those who did not participate in agenda preparation

More than 170 government delegations participated in negotiating *Agenda 21*. To the extent that governments can provide an accurate reflection of the wishes and concerns of the populations they represent, the majority of the world's population was at least represented in the discussions which led to *Agenda 21*. Government delegations included senior-level civil servants and, in some cases, government-sponsored special advisers on environmental issues and/or representatives of non-governmental environment and development organizations. As stated earlier, the majority of government representatives came from environment or national resource ministries rather than from ministries for business, industry, trade, commerce or finance. The participation of NGOs in the preparation of government statements was at a level never achieved during previous UN conferences.

During the final two PREPCOM meetings various groups, usually organized around other than national affiliation such as environment NGOs and development NGOs, began pressing for amendments to government statements and to chapters within *Agenda 21*. Many of the NGOs which prepared agendas were politically very sophisticated with experience of lobbying in the international arena. International organizations of women, youth, indigenous peoples and local governments, including most of the groups which prepared the agendas compared here, were present at the PREPCOMS pressing for changes to the existing text of *Agenda 21*. This required persuading government delegations to introduce the desired changes during negotiations of *Agenda 21*. There is a general consensus that women's groups were the most effective in obtaining additions to the text of *Agenda 21* that reflect the problems and potential solutions facing women in the area of environment and development. In the final version of *Agenda 21* the role of women or the problems facing women are specifically mentioned in all except seven chapters.[22]

From among international groups labour unions were not particularly involved in lobbying to alter the content of *Agenda 21*. While the media was actively covering many of the events relating to UNCED they did not participate in developing or altering *Agenda 21* text. A number of religious groups took part in the UNCED process (such as the International Co-ordinating Committee on Religion and the Earth) but they tended to place greater emphasis on the creation of an Earth Charter than on *Agenda 21*.

The working documents from which *Agenda 21* eventually emerged were in English, although translations in at least French and Spanish were usually also available. However, this meant that those who were able to work in English often had the greatest ease in reading and responding to informal and formal proposed changes. Those dependent on non-European languages such as Arabic, Mandarin or Hindi would have had some difficulty in obtaining translations of the rapid changes to the text that occurred as the Earth Summit approached.

The language barrier in international negotiations is often less of a factor than it might seem, both because for UN-facilitated negotiations high-quality interpretation and translation are readily available and because the vast majority of those participating in international work are often able to work in English or are bilingual, with English, Spanish or French as a second language.

The language issue highlights the fact that it is generally the privileged who take part in any capacity in international negotiations – privileged in terms of education and the ability to travel outside their own country. Using this definition, more people from developed countries are likely to participate in international meetings or lobbying activities. And generally, although not always, participants from developing countries come from a relatively elite group within their own society. To put it bluntly, there is little chance that the world's poor, oppressed, discouraged or over-stressed had any reasonable level of input into *Agenda 21*, although some NGOs attempted to represent this component of world society.

The intended users

The agendas are full of suggestions, recommendations and, in some cases, warnings, directed at a wide variety of actors including different levels of government, ministries, international financial institutions and professional associations.

The vast majority of recommendations in all the agendas were directed at national governments. This is natural, both because the main event was a United Nations Conference and because national governments have access to the human, financial, technical and other types of resources needed to realize change.

Agenda Ya Wananchi, *Caring for the Earth*, the *Women's Action Agenda*, the *Youth Action Guide on Sustainable Development* and *Voice of the Eagle* also consistently directed recommendation to local governments or communities. The two sector-specific agendas discussed here, *ASCEND 21* and *Changing Course*, addressed a number of recommendations to the different levels of government but concentrated on the roles that their constituencies could play in supporting forward movement on sustainability.

3

ECONOMIC CONSIDERATIONS

The concept of sustainable development is based on the assumption that all types of human activity are interrelated. In 'sustainability-speak', this is usually expressed as 'the importance of integrating social, economic and environmental objectives into planning, decision-making and implementation of projects and programmes'.

In this chapter, we examine how the various agendas tackle economic issues. Table 3.1 illustrates the economic issues considered by the agendas. The difficulty of looking at this or any area in isolation reflects the fact that a sustainable approach to economics must, by definition, also take into account the social and ecological aspects of a problem. Some of the material in this and the next two chapters overlaps, demonstrating that we are dealing with complex and connected issues.

Table 3.1 Economic issues covered in the agendas

	Business & industry	Consumption	Poverty	Trade, debt
Agenda 21	✓	✓	✓	✓
NGO Alternative Treaties	✓	✓	✓	✓
Agenda Ya Wananchi	✗	✗	✓	✓
ASCEND 21	✗	✓	✗	✗
Caring for the Earth	✓	✓	✗	✗
Women's Action Agenda 21	✗	✓	✓	✓
Global Assembly of Women and the Environment	✗	✗	✗	✗
Youth '92	✗	✗	✓	✓
Youth Action Guide	✓	✗	✗	✓
Voice of the Eagle	✗	✗	✗	✗
Changing Course	✓	✗	✓	✓

✓ = major priority area   ✗ = not a major priority area

Many of the thorny problems of implementing sustainability are linked to economic conditions, in particular the equitable distribution of economic assets.

Major topics covered in this chapter include business and industry, consumption, poverty, and trade and debt. There is a brief overview of the key points relating to sustainability in these areas, followed by a discussion of how they are treated within and between agendas.

The pursuit of economic growth is one of the fundamental principles of the current approach to development – and one of the more divisive issues among the agendas. There is a yawning gulf between those who accept that the current approach is flawed but believe that it can be repaired, and the others who insist that we would be better off discarding the whole thing and starting over. Issues such as trade, debt, market mechanisms and income and lifestyle disparities between rich and poor are hotly contested across the agendas.

Business and industry

Proposals about business and industry were made in the following agendas:

Agenda 21   chapter 30: Strengthening and Role of Business and Industry

NGO Alternative Treaties   Treaty on Transnational Corporations: Democratic Regulation of their Conduct

Caring for the Earth   chapter 11: Business, Industry and Commerce

Youth Action Guide   chapter 9: Industry and Environment

Changing Course   chapter 1: The Business of Sustainable Development

The major players in business and industry are sometimes seen as both the villains and the potential heroes of the sustainable development movement. This is particularly true of large multinational companies. The *NGO Alternative Treaty on Transnational Corporations* calls TNCs among 'the main actors in the global environmental crisis' and blames them for perpetuating 'social and political inequality and loss of cultural diversity'. On the other hand, the role of the private sector is repeatedly cited as important for attaining sustainable development. This is the case in *Agenda 21* and in the more recent *Programme for the Further Implementation of Agenda 21*, which states that 'the investment, role and the responsibilities of business and industry, including transnational corporations, are important'.[23]

Major points of comparison among the agendas

Agenda 21 and the *NGO Alternative Treaty* take very different approaches to the private sector. *Agenda 21* makes a wide-ranging recommendation for business and industry to become cleaner and more efficient, while the *NGO Treaty on Transnational Corporations* narrows in on what signatories call 'the role of transnational corporations in the global environmental crisis'. *Agenda*

16

21 encourages TNCs to establish corporate policies on sustainable development including 'responsible and ethical management of products and
processes', actions that are largely to be undertaken through self-regulation.
The *NGO Alternative Treaty*, on the other hand, is adamant about the need for
TNCs to be monitored and regulated from outside and accused UNCED of
having 'abdicated its responsibility to take measures to control TNC
activities'.

Caring for the Earth, like *Agenda 21*, cites the need for improving efficiency
in production and increasing the use of clean technologies. However, these
recommendations come within the framework of businesses operating
according to an 'ethic for living sustainably' which is not mentioned in
Agenda 21. *Caring for the Earth* also provides specific guidelines for regulating the operations of business and industry (for example, adoption of the
polluter-pays principle) and encourages governments to develop more effective legislation to control practices such as packaging and disposal of
hazardous substances. *Agenda 21* places greater weight on increasing self-
regulation.

There are several similarities between *Agenda 21*, which focuses on the need
for more efficient production, and the *Youth Action Guide* with its broader
appeal for business to work towards achieving sustainable development and a
list of reasons why this is necessary (such as current short-term planning rather
than life-cycle analysis, industrial production of toxic waste, lack of industry
standards). Both documents propose including workers and unions in programme development and training for operations that promote the objectives
of sustainable development. The *Youth Action Guide* emphasizes controlling
industry (for example, issuing permits on the basis of acceptable pollution
levels, heavily taxing environmentally harmful products) while at the same
time suggesting self-regulation and encouraging multinational corporations to
take the lead.

Five years later

The World Business Council for Sustainable Development (WBCSD) has done
considerable follow-up on many of the recommendations in *Changing Course*.
This is well documented in its 1997 publication *Signals of Change*, in which it
states, 'much has been achieved; much more has begun; and much remains
ahead of us'. Examples of these initiatives appear in Chapter 7. The current
executive director of WBCSD states: 'I wish that all parts of society were
changing as quickly and as much as industry'.[24]

There has been a long-running debate within the sustainable development
community about whether industry should be regulated or encouraged to
develop voluntary standards. So while the WBCSD has identified its own
examples of improvement there are those who feel that more impartial monitoring of business activities needs to be undertaken. As Peter Padbury, a key

organizer of the International NGO Forum which drove the *NGO Alternative Treaty* process in Rio, observed:

> Although NGOs are happy that terms like eco-efficiency are now included in business literature, many are very unhappy with the collapse of government capacity to monitor and enforce regulations. The move towards voluntary compliance could become a new battleground. Independent environmental audits by trustworthy firms, paid for by the corporation and reporting to the public, could help to give credibility and accountability to corporate 'volunteerism'.[25]

Other NGOs, such as the Women's Environment and Development Organization, believe business has yet to go far enough. According to WEDO, as a rule the private sector and large private sector entities do not yet take the post-Rio agenda seriously, and it is these very entities that remain, to a large extent, outside the control of NGOs, civil society, even at times of their own stakeholders.[26]

Consumption

Agenda 21	chapter 4: Changing Consumption Patterns
NGO Alternative Treaties	Treaty on Consumption and Lifestyle
ASCEND 21	chapter 12: Quality of Life
Caring for the Earth	chapter 5: Keeping within the Earth's Carrying Capacity
Women's Action Agenda 21	Women's Consumer Power

Unsustainable patterns of consumption and production, particularly in the North, were cited a number of times throughout *Agenda 21* as one of the driving forces behind existing unsustainable conditions.

Consumption is approached from different angles by agendas that identify the issue as a priority. Some emphasize the inequities (*Women's Action Agenda 21*) and the social imbalances (*Agenda 21*) caused by current patterns of consumption. The *Women's Action Agenda 21* and the *NGO Treaty on Consumption and Lifestyle* link serious environmental degradation and development problems to prevailing consumption practices. *Caring for the Earth* focuses on keeping human population and demand for resources within the Earth's carrying capacity, while *ASCEND 21* asks what researchers can do to improve the quality of life.

The reasons for consumption-related problems include excessive demand for resources such as energy, water and minerals, particularly from the rich (*Agenda 21*, *Caring for the Earth*, *ASCEND 21*). Here the rich are considered to be the majority in upper-income countries and the elite in poorer countries. The *Women's Action Agenda 21* cites current policies and spending choices which encourage consumption at the expense of environmental protection and social equity. The *NGO Alternative Treaty* concurs with the *Women's Action Agenda 21* but is more specific in criticizing the present 'world economic order' which 'exhausts and contaminates natural resources and creates and perpetuates gross inequalities between and within nations'.

Major points of comparison among the agendas

The major difference between *Agenda 21* and the *NGO Alternative Treaty* lies in what they consider appropriate action. *Agenda 21* concentrates on measures at the national and regional level while the NGOs stress the need for a personal commitment to change and for clearer values throughout society. The *NGO Alternative Treaty* also identifies a broader reason for current unsustainable consumption and lifestyle patterns – the 'world economic order'.

ASCEND 21 frames the question from the more specific perspective of the contribution researchers can make towards improving the quality of life globally, including altering unsustainable consumption and production patterns. The science agenda pushes further into the theoretical realm, suggesting multidisciplinary research on issues such as understanding the meaning of 'quality of life' with respect to human needs.

Agenda 21 and *Caring for the Earth* define the main consumption problem differently. *Caring for the Earth* identifies the Earth's carrying capacity as the factor ultimately limiting consumption, while *Agenda 21* stops at recognizing current unsustainable consumption practices. Both documents state that unsustainable lifestyles among the rich in developed and developing countries are the principal cause of over-consumption. *Caring for the Earth* adds that the situation is exacerbated by existing conditions where the rich control the mechanisms for changing the distribution of wealth. Most of the actions proposed in response to over-consumption are the same.

The *Women's Action Agenda 21* maintains that over-consumption is made worse by policies that do not give priority to environmental protection and social equity. Proposed activities to reduce consumption and waste include more efficient production of goods, recycling and lifestyle changes such as reducing the use of cars in favour of public transport.

The United Nations General Assembly Special Session on progress since the Earth Summit concluded that, 'while unsustainable patterns in the industrialised countries continue to aggravate the threats to the environment, there remain huge difficulties for developing countries in meeting basic needs such as food, health care, shelter and education for people'. Indicators of consumption such as fossil fuel use show consumption of non-renewable fuels and the associated emissions at an all-time high in 1996.[27] In spite of the recommendations made in the various agendas, consumption and production levels have not yet begun to decline.

Poverty

Agenda 21	chapter 3: Combating Poverty
NGO Alternative Treaties	Poverty Treaty
Agenda Ya Wananchi	Appeal to Governments: Launch a Major Anti-poverty Campaign
Women's Action Agenda 21	Women, Poverty, Land Rights, Food Security and Credit
Youth '92	Poverty
Changing Course	chapter 10: Leadership for Sustainable Development in Developing Countries

Poverty is often defined as the lack of access to adequate basic resources such as food, shelter, energy, education and clothing.

All eleven agendas under consideration include poverty as an important issue. The six agendas which make poverty a priority define it as a lack of means to obtain the physical essentials of daily living. *Youth '92* and the *NGO Poverty Treaty* both point out poverty's negative effects on the mental and spiritual well-being of individuals, and *Youth '92* criticizes the fact that poverty is so often defined in economic terms only.

The main causes of poverty are identified as the inequity of current income distribution and unequal access to needed resources (*Agenda 21*, *Youth '92*, *Women's Action Agenda 21*, *NGO Alternative Treaties*). *Women's Action Agenda 21* and *Youth '92* highlight the fact that more women than men are denied access to basic needs. *Youth '92* also blames 'the military industry' and 'unfair and unequal policies in international trade and political decision-making'. *Changing Course* sees a link between poverty and 'the movement of families to unsuitable areas'.

Major points of comparison among the agendas

The *NGO Alternative Treaty* focuses on several basic and broad solutions to world poverty, while *Agenda 21* recommends a country-by-country approach. The two documents agree on the importance of community and local action and on the urgent need to assist the most disadvantaged groups – women, children, farmers, artisans, fishing communities and indigenous peoples. Debt is another topic raised in both documents: NGOs propose cancelling the external debt of poor countries; *Agenda 21* recognizes the relationship between environmental/social degradation and external debt but is vague about a solution. *Agenda Ya Wananchi* appeals to all governments to undertake a 'major anti-poverty programme' funded by a consumption tax on the rich.

Poverty alleviation and food security are important issues in the *Women's Action Agenda 21* although here, naturally enough, they are considered specifically from the perspective of women and the particular prejudices that limit women's access to necessary resources. *Agenda 21* proposes increasing the equity of income distribution (chapters 3 and 14) but does not address this in gender terms. *Agenda 21* recognizes a connection between promoting economic growth in developing countries and enhanced food security. The *Women's Action Agenda 21* stresses that in many societies where women bear the main responsibility for providing food to the family unit they require equal access to resources such as land and development assistance (such as land ownership, land inheritance). *Agenda 21* links food scarcity with population growth. This issue is not raised in the *Women's Action Agenda 21*.

Youth '92 states that current international trade policies, the military industry, the unequal status of women and the management of local resources by governments and multinational corporations are the primary forces preventing people from meeting their basic requirements for living.

Agenda 21 and *Changing Course* consider poverty differently. *Agenda 21* focuses on unfair income distribution and poor development of human resources, while *Changing Course* highlights the poverty which results from increasing urbanization due to policies and programmes that place the urban dweller at a disadvantage economically and socially.

Five years later there is little evidence that progress has been made on the alleviation of poverty. A recent study by the Bangladesh Centre for Advanced Studies[28] concluded that 'the over-consumption of the North and rampant poverty in the South remain the greatest threats to the attainment of the sustainable global development'. The United Nations General Assembly Special Session reported that

> the five years since the Rio Conference have witnessed an increase in the number of people living in absolute poverty, particularly in developing countries. In this context, there is an urgent need for the timely and full implementation of all the relevant commitments, agreements and targets already agreed upon since the Rio Conference by the international community, including the United Nations system and international financial institutions. Full implementation of the Programme of Action of the World Summit for Social Development is essential.

Trade and debt

Agenda 21	chapter 2: International Co-operation to Accelerate Sustainable Development in Developing Countries and Related Domestic Policies
NGO Alternative Treaties	Alternative Treaty on Trade and Sustainable Development, Debt Treaty
Agenda Ya Wananchi	NGO Commitment 11 – Promote Alternative

	Trade; Appeal to Governments – Reduce Debt Burden in Central and Eastern Europe and in the South; Reform the World Trading System
Women's Action Agenda 21	Foreign Debt and Trade
Youth '92	External Debt
Youth Action Guide	chapter 11: International Trade
Changing Course	chapter 5: Trade and Sustainable Development; chapter 10: Leadership for Sustainable Development in Developing Countries

The primary differences among the agendas which address trade and debt concern whether existing models of development based on economic growth serve the greatest number of people while furthering the goals of environmental protection and equitable social development.

The issues of trade and debt are linked as international monetary issues in most of the agendas. *Youth '92* concentrates on debt and *Agenda 21* raises these topics as major programme areas in a chapter which gives the impression that trade and debt are areas where developed countries need to help developing ones.

The majority of agendas express concern about current world trading practices. For some, they are 'not socially just or ecologically sustainable' (*NGO Alternative Treaties*, *Youth '92*), are dominated by a few privileged players such as governments of developed countries or TNCs (*Agenda Ya Wananchi*, *Youth '92*), or are hindered by imposed economic barriers such as tariffs and import quotas (*Changing Course*). The *Women's Action Agenda 21* says that present trade and debt situations perpetuate poor economic conditions in developing countries, while *Agenda 21* identifies the problem, rather vaguely, as the difficulty of integrating the goals of environment and development.

Various reasons are put forward for trade problems and heavy foreign debt, including an unfair development model which leads to the South subsidizing the rich countries of the North (*Women's Action Agenda 21*, *NGO Alternative Treaties*, *Agenda Ya Wananchi*, *Youth '92*) and greed (*Youth Action Guide*). According to the *Youth Action Guide* and *Changing Course*, problems also result, in part, from market manipulation such as protectionism and heavy subsidization of certain sectors of the economy (such as agriculture) by governments. The *Women's Action Agenda 21* and *Youth '92* point to the negative impacts of World Bank and IMF structural adjustment programmes. *Changing Course* supports these as possible solutions to the debt problem.

The greatest controversy regarding trade and debt revolves around whether the current development model, with a few changes, is adequate for achieving goals such as fair trade or reduced disparities, or whether a completely new approach is required. The agendas which address trade and debt are divided on this issue. *Agenda 21*, the *Youth Action Guide* and *Changing Course* favour modifications to the existing system, while the *NGO Alternative Treaties*, *Agenda Ya*

Wananchi, the *Women's Action Agenda 21* and *Youth '92* are very critical of current approaches to development.

Major points of comparison among the agendas

The *NGO Alternative Treaties* and *Agenda 21* diverge widely on trade and debt issues. The problems are not even defined in the same way. *Agenda 21* does attempt to identify the underlying cause of the problem, while NGOs cite the current 'predatory model of development' and the 'indebtedness of the Southern countries'. *Agenda 21* argues that sustainable development may be enhanced through the success of agreements such as GATT, while the *NGO Alternative Treaties* regard these agreements as being in the corporate rather than the public interest and call for the formation of a new International Trade Organization based on equity. It should be remembered that these agendas were written before the advent of the World Trade Organization.

Agenda Ya Wananchi also differs from *Agenda 21* on the issues of trade and debt. *Agenda 21* emphasizes the difficulty, and the necessity, of integrating the goals of environment and development to work towards sustainable development. *Agenda Ya Wananchi* blames unfair trading systems for current trade and debt problems. The various actions recommended in the two documents reflect these different interpretations, with *Agenda 21* looking towards the liberalization of trade and compatible national government policies on environment and development. The two agendas agree that developing countries need more resources, but *Agenda Ya Wananchi* goes on to state that this is mainly because of international trade policies which produce 'a net transfer of financial resources from the poor to the rich'. *Agenda Ya Wananchi* declares a commitment to alternative and fair trade, and advocates that citizens and those governing them should work towards changing the current trading system (including taking into account environmental concerns during trade negotiations).

Agenda 21 addresses the issues of trade and debt within the context of the difficulty of integrating environmental and development goals. The *Women's Action Agenda 21* focuses on the consequences of social and environmental problems with a special acknowledgement of the issues facing women. The agendas disagree on remedial action. The *Women's Action Agenda 21* calls for the cancellation of foreign debt, while *Agenda 21* states, more generally, the need to provide adequate financial resources to developing countries.

Youth '92, noting the economic inequality between North and South resulting from colonization, the programmes of international financial institutions and high foreign debt, also proposes cancelling the foreign debt of developing countries, a policy not mentioned in *Agenda 21*.

Agenda 21 and the *Youth Action Guide* recognize the interrelated nature of environment and development and emphasize the link between increased trade liberalization and better environmental management. The *Youth Action*

Guide proposes self-restructuring by multinational corporations to allow for more local decision-making. Both documents propose reducing and rescheduling the foreign debt of developing countries under conditions such as accepting terms of economic adjustment policies (*Agenda 21*) or debt-for-nature exchanges (*Youth Action Guide*).

While *Agenda 21* identifies the broad objective of integrating environmental and development goals, *Changing Course* homes in on current obstacles to development and environmental compatibility. Apart from this initial difference in perspective, many of the recommendations of *Agenda 21* and *Changing Course* are similar, including trade liberalization, clarifying the role of GATT in environmental matters and using economic structural adjustment programmes to reduce debt. *Agenda 21* counsels caution with this last activity in the light of 'adverse social and environmental effects' in some countries. The potential negative aspects of certain types of macroeconomic reforms are not addressed in this chapter of *Changing Course*.

Five years after these agendas were written, various reports on trade and sustainability have reached a similar conclusion: everyone is talking about trade and sustainable development, or at least about trade's impact on the environment, but nobody is doing much about it. 'The Commission on Sustainable Development has called three times for development of a framework to assess the environmental impacts of trade and investment policy,' says the World Wildlife Fund's Charles Arden-Clarke in his report on trade globalization.[29] 'It is generating paper once a year, but it is not generating actions. Meanwhile, the World Trade Organisation is essentially paralysed on the issue . . . increasing rather than decreasing the potential for conflict between multilateral trade agreements and environmental regimes.' According to the International Institute for Sustainable Development,[30] the WTO and GATT before it have made little progress on issues of environmental openness and there is a critical need to expand the focus of debate from trade and environment to trade, environment *and* development.

Five years after the Earth Summit, UNGASS reported that

> the external debt problem continues to hamper the efforts of developing countries to achieve sustainable development. To resolve the remaining debt problems of the heavily indebted poor countries, creditor and debtor countries and international financial institutions should continue their efforts to find effective, equitable, development oriented and durable solutions to the debt problem.

4

SOCIAL DEVELOPMENT

Social development refers to how well societies are meeting basic human needs such as food, shelter and clothing. It also involves providing the support services that can make or break the quality of a life, including health care, education, culture and human rights. In this chapter social development issues are examined within the context of sustainable development.

Integrating social development with wise ecological management and sustainable economic development is seen as vital for achieving sustainability. Table 4.1 shows the social development issues addressed by the different agendas. The discussion of each topic includes an introduction, a summary of the differences between and among the agendas, a more detailed presentation of the points of comparison and a summary of what has happened in these areas since the Earth Summit.

Capacity building

Agenda 21	chapter 37: Capacity Building in Developing Countries
ASCEND 21	chapter 14: Capacity Building
Caring for the Earth	chapter 9: Creating a Global Alliance

Capacity building generally describes efforts that develop an ability to achieve goals. Building capacity to implement sustainability depends on available knowledge and the ability to adapt and act upon this knowledge where it is needed. Most often capacity building is achieved through training, public participation, network building and exchange programmes.

Three agendas focus on capacity building within the framework of environment and development. *Agenda 21* considers capacity building for policy development and evaluation 'keeping in mind environmental potentials and limits and needs as perceived by the people'. *ASCEND 21* highlights the capacity building needed in adjusting to change and the implementation of *Agenda 21*. *Caring for the Earth* emphasizes the need for capacity building in low-income countries in order to increase economic prosperity, sustainable development and environmental protection.

Table 4.1 Social issues covered in the agendas

	Capacity building	Children	Decision-making	Democracy	Education	Ethics, Values	Health	Indigenous peoples	Institutions	Local initiatives	Military	Population	NGOs	Urbanization	Women
Agenda 21	✓	✓	✓	✗	✓	✗	✓	✓	✓	✓	✗	✓	✓	✓	✓
NGO Alternative Treaties	✗	✓	✓	✗	✓	✓	✗	✓	✗	✗	✓	✓	✓	✓	✓
Agenda Ya Wananchi	✗	✗	✗	✓	✓	✓	✗	✓	✓	✗	✓	✗	✗	✓	✓
ASCEND 21	✓	✗	✗	✗	✓	✗	✓	✗	✓	✗	✗	✓	✗	✗	✗
Caring for the Earth	✓	✗	✗	✗	✓	✓	✓	✗	✗	✓	✗	✓	✗	✓	✗
Women's Action Agenda 21	✗	✗	✗	✓	✓	✓	✓	✗	✗	✗	✗	✓	✗	✗	✓
Global Assembly of Women and the Environment	✗	✗	✗	✗	✗	✗	✗	✗	✗	✗	✗	✗	✗	✗	✓
Youth '92	✗	✗	✗	✓	✗	✗	✗	✗	✗	✗	✓	✗	✗	✓	✓
Youth Action Guide	✗	✓	✗	✓	✓	✗	✓	✓	✓	✗	✓	✓	✗	✗	✗
Voice of the Eagle	✗	✓	✗	✗	✓	✓	✓	✗	✗	✗	✗	✗	✗	✓	✓
Changing Course	✗	✗	✗	✗	✓	✗	✗	✗	✗	✗	✗	✓	✗	✗	✗

✓ = a major priority area   ✗ = not a major area

Major points of comparison among the agendas

Agenda 21 stresses the importance of building and improving capacity based on what the people concerned consider to be important. *ASCEND 21's* approach is to improve methods for transferring skills and knowledge and to find ways to help individuals respond to a changing world. *Agenda 21* is primarily concerned with capacity building to implement *Agenda 21*. *ASCEND 21* acknowledges the value of implementing *Agenda 21* along with the agenda for the scientific community. Both documents propose actions to strengthen institutions and co-operation among institutions while encouraging local participation, training and infrastructure development.

Caring for the Earth considers capacity building with respect to developing countries. For *Agenda 21*, this means focusing on the role of people and institutions at the national level, while *Caring for the Earth* emphasizes interdependence among nations and trade and debt inequities for developed countries.

Five years later

Following UNCED, the United Nations Commission on Sustainable Development (CSD) was set up to oversee national governments' implementation of *Agenda 21*. Some initial confusion arose regarding the separate roles of the CSD and the United Nations Environment Programme. This is in part a reflection of the mistaken view that the single most important component of sustainable development is the environment. The United Nations Development Programme continues to be the international agency with the strongest mandate to support capacity building for the implementation of *Agenda 21*. The roles of these different agencies are clarified in the UNGASS report which states: 'the role of UNEP, as the principal United Nations body in the field of environment, should be enhanced. . . . UNEP is to be the leading global environmental authority that sets the environmental dimension of sustainable development within the United Nations'. And 'UNDP should continue to strengthen its contribution to and programmes in sustainable development and the implementation of *Agenda 21* at all levels particularly in the area of promoting capacity-building, in co-operation with other organisations, as well as in the field of poverty eradication'.

These distinctions in duties, while logical, indicate a tendency to continue to separate the environment and development issues which underlie sustainability.

Children

Agenda 21   chapter 25: Children and Youth in Sustainable Development

27

NGO Alternative Treaties	Treaty in Defence and Protection of Children and Adolescents, Youth Treaty
Voice of the Eagle	Children of the Creator

Two of the agendas that consider children in the context of environment and development focus on the effects of environmental degradation on children. The third (*Voice of the Eagle*) expresses the belief that environmental degradation results from the failure to teach children that they are part of the natural environment. *Agenda 21* highlights children's vulnerability in the face of environmental deterioration. The *NGO Treaty in Defence and Protection of Children and Adolescents* maintains that a decline in environmental quality violates the fundamental rights of children and adolescents.

The *NGO Alternative Treaty* points to an international development model that promotes social inequality and environmental degradation as well as an inequitable relationship between North and South caused by 'the politics of domination and discrimination'. *Agenda 21* does not attempt to explain the causes of environmental degradation. It does look at the contributions young people can make towards improving the relationship between environment and development and also considers the vulnerability of children to human rights abuses and environmental problems. This is very different from *Voice of the Eagle*, which stresses, instead, the need to raise children with an awareness of their relationship with the environment and their part in the natural world.

The *Youth Treaty* begins by denouncing the lack of concrete responses from UNCED to global dilemmas and how they impact on youth and children. However, the activities proposed by the *NGO Alternative Treaties* and *Agenda 21* (for example, increasing participation of the young in environment and development decision-making, improving access to education) are very similar to the recommendations of the *Youth Treaty*.

Five years later

In a report evaluating youth participation in the implementation of sustainability as outlined in *Agenda 21*, Peace Child International states:

> By endorsing the idea of partnership in all these declarations and summit statements, governments signal their commitments to a more active, and equal, responsibility to citizenship for disenfranchised young people . . . [but it is possible] to demonstrate how far short of that commitment governments, the UN and its agencies and most other institutions have fallen.

Decision-making

Agenda 21	chapter 8: Integrating Environment and

28

| | Development in Decision-making; chapter 40: Information for Decision-making |
| *NGO Alternative Treaties* | Rio Framework Treaty on NGO Global Decision-making |

Only two of the eleven documents put special emphasis on decision-making, although three agendas which focus on democracy (*ASCEND 21*, *Women's Action Agenda 21*, *Youth '92*) raise some of the same issues.

Major points of comparison between the agendas

The *NGO Alternative Treaties* and the relevant chapters in *Agenda 21* express very similar ideas about decision-making. *Agenda 21* provides more concrete suggestions for action by governments (such as review of policies) while the NGOs' priority is to increase their own effectiveness in the decision-making process by improving their networks and enhancing current levels of reporting and co-ordination.

Democracy

Agenda Ya Wananchi	NGO Commitment: Expand Participatory Democracy, Appeal to Governments: Enhance and Promote Participatory Democracy
Women's Action Agenda 21	Democratic Rights, Diversity, Solidarity
Youth '92	Democracy and Participation

All eleven agendas emphasize the need for greater participation in decision-making at various levels and on a large number of issues. Three agendas have separate sections which specifically address democracy. *Youth '92* and *Agenda Ya Wananchi* consider democracy and participation, while the *Women's Action Agenda 21* looks at democratic rights, diversity and solidarity. Informed and representative participation are the two major areas considered. Sections of other agendas dealing with education, awareness and access to information overlap with many of the issues raised here.

Youth '92 defines democracy as a 'tool for social transformation' and outlines how, depending upon the context, democracy takes many forms including social, political and economic. *Agenda Ya Wananchi* states that 'people's participation is the ultimate guarantee of justice and sustainability' and calls on all governments to 'enhance and promote participatory democracy in all issues and at all levels'. *Women's Action Agenda 21* observes that women and other groups traditionally are not represented in decision-making bodies in contravention of their democratic rights.

Five years later

Democracy illustrated by broadened participation in decision-making continues to be cited as an important component of achieving sustainability
throughout all review-of-progress documents put forward for the Earth
Summit +5.

Education

Agenda 21	chapter 36: Promoting Education Public Awareness and Training
NGO Alternative Treaties	Treaty on Environmental Education for Sustainable Societies and Global Responsibility
Agenda Ya Wananchi	NGO Commitment 13: Educate People on the Importance of Cultural Diversity
ASCEND 21	chapter 13: Public Awareness, Science and the Environment
Caring for the Earth	chapter 6: Changing Personal Attitudes and Practices
Women's Action Agenda 21	Information and Education
Youth Action Guide	chapter 16: Education
Voice of the Eagle	Awareness
Changing Course	chapter 10: Leadership for Sustainable Development in Developing Countries

Education (along with the related issues of awareness and information) is the
topic addressed by the largest number of agendas – nine out of eleven. Slightly
different types of education are called for in each agenda, highlighting the variety of perspectives these documents bring to the most pressing environment
and development issues. However, although the educational needs that are
addressed vary, they do not necessarily conflict, and the value of considering a
problem from more than one perspective is amply illustrated.

Four agendas call for more education but with a slightly different focus.
Agenda 21 raises the need for education in all areas required to implement
Agenda 21. *Changing Course* states there is a need to educate in all issues relating to sustainable development. The *NGO Alternative Treaty on Environmental
Education* sees a need to educate for the changes required to achieve equitable
sustainability. And *Caring for the Earth* considers education in light of the
changes necessary to achieve sustainable living. These educational goals illustrate the different priorities of the various groups which can be found
throughout the agendas.

The *NGO Alternative Treaty* focuses on equity and sustainability, omitting the
word 'development'. *Caring for the Earth* also avoids development in order to
focus on the type of education needed for societies to change personal lifestyle

and consumption and live sustainably. *Agenda 21* and *Changing Course* stress the need to harness education to achieve the goals of sustainable development.

The goal of increasing awareness is mentioned in several agendas but often with a slightly different meaning. In *Agenda 21* it means public awareness while in *Voice of the Eagle* it is spiritual awareness, as in 'an awareness of the balance of all natural life'. *ASCEND 21*, meanwhile, poses the question: what contribution can and should science make towards the development of public awareness of environmental problems? The need for more information for better decision-making is another theme which runs through the *Youth Action Guide* and the *Women's Action Agenda 21*.

The various attitudes towards educational goals and needs reflect, at least in part, the underlying values and priorities in the documents. For the *NGO Alternative Treaties*, equity and sustainability must go hand in hand. But this emphasis on equity is not found, for example, in *Changing Course*. Education is a sensitive area. One group's idea of what constitutes education may be seen by another group as an attempt to reinforce the status quo or to indoctrinate from the perspective of an unrealistic world-view. Note the reasons given by the *NGO Alternative Treaty* and the *Youth Action Guide* as to why changes in approaches to education are needed. The *NGO Treaty on Environmental Education for Sustainable Societies and Global Responsibility* cites the current socio-economic system based on over-consumption for some and under-consumption and inadequate conditions for production for the majority. The *Youth Action Guide* points to *inappropriate* (italics added) education policies that omit education on subjects such as human rights or humanitarian concerns.

Major points of comparison among the agendas

Once again, *Agenda 21* and the *NGO Alternative Treaties* differ markedly in the way they perceive the problem. *Agenda 21* focuses on increasing awareness and education in order to further the goals of *Agenda 21*, while the *NGO Alternative Treaty* seeks to educate for achieving sustainability including enhanced awareness of the problems associated with the dominant socio-economic system. The actual activities proposed (for example, education and training that is interdisciplinary and democratic) are very similar with the exception of the NGOs' commitment to work together.

Agenda Ya Wananchi stresses the importance of increasing awareness and educating on issues relating to cultural diversity. Both are within the scope of *Agenda 21* but *Ya Wananchi* gives them much more weight. Both documents highlight the need for changes in society but the dissimilarity in educational goals is reflected in the actions proposed for achieving those changes.

One of the major differences between *ASCEND 21* and *Agenda 21* is the way they address the issue of education and science. *Agenda 21* emphasizes the role scientists can play in providing information for decision-making on environment and development policy, while *ASCEND 21* states that scientists need to

31

clarify their role in raising awareness of environmental problems. The activities proposed in the two main chapters on education and science illustrate this difference in perspective. The role of science, as stated in chapter 14 (Capacity Building) of *ASCEND 21*, is closer to the more traditional discussion of the contribution that the scientific community can make by sharing knowledge and increasing participation in decision-making.

Caring for the Earth places greater emphasis on changing personal attitudes and practices than *Agenda 21*, which, as noted above, focuses on education and training for implementing *Agenda 21*, a document which explores institutional and government approaches to sustainable development more fully than personal commitment to change. *Caring for the Earth* suggests strategies for increasing personal awareness and knowledge (for instance, non-formal education and communication such as parental influence). While *Agenda 21* also recognizes the need for non-formal communication, it takes a closer look at training to achieve specific sustainable development goals as articulated in *Agenda 21* (such as training of aid agency workers to increase awareness of those activities which are environmentally sound and those which are not). This is, however, one of the few chapters in *Agenda 21* where the spiritual aspects of environment and development are raised.

The *Women's Action Agenda 21* also raises a number of topics which either do not appear or are covered briefly in *Agenda 21*, including the environmental and health impacts of military activity and the importance of educating on cultural diversity and integrity.

The *Youth Action Guide* looks at education and 'improving the quality of life'. From this perspective, *Agenda 21* proposes activities to enhance awareness of environment and development issues, while the *Youth Action Guide* favours education on human rights, humanitarian concerns and increasing public participation in the media.

Agenda 21 deals with raising awareness of the interaction between humans and the natural world in technical terms such as changes in policies and programmes, *Voice of the Eagle* encourages the use of the senses to increase awareness of the balance of all natural life. *Voice of the Eagle* begins with the premise that all changes must come from 'a deep reverence for the sanctity of all life' and an 'awareness of the balance of all life'.

Changing Course and *Agenda 21* both stress the importance of training to obtain the required skills for achieving sustainable development. *Agenda 21* takes a broad view of the type of education needed, while *Changing Course* looks more specifically at business, industry, engineering and management of technology.

Five years later

In 1997, many of the education recommendations remain unrealized. Global Education Associates' Project Global 2000 reports[31] that there

is an urgent need to move the education goals of *Agenda 21* from articulation and agreement to local, national and international action. It is
somewhat clear that all parties see the importance of education for
sustainable development. It is not clear how well this concept is
understood and why it receives such low political and economic priority at the national and international levels.

Ethics, values

NGO Alternative Treaties	Ethical Commitments to Global Ecological Posture and Behaviour
Agenda Ya Wananchi	Preamble, The Current World Order
Caring for the Earth	Foreword, Building a Sustainable Society
Women's Action Agenda 21	Code of Environmental Ethics and Accountability

Ethics deals with what is right or wrong, good or bad. Therefore, all the agendas in this book ascribe, directly or indirectly, to a certain ethical point of view.
Even if they are not presented in a separate section, statements regarding
ethics and values can be found throughout the agendas. *Youth '92*, for example,
tells us that youth of the South should fight the infiltration of Western consumer values. *Agenda 21*, chapter 30, states that business and industry
including TNCs should ensure responsible and ethical management of products and processes.

The primary difference among agendas on ethics and values is that a number
of them stress the importance of working from an ethical framework on environment and development problems (*Agenda Ya Wananchi*, *Caring for the Earth*,
the *Women's Action Agenda 21*, *Voice of the Eagle*) while others do not explicitly
address this issue. Instead, they demonstrate values through problem definition and proposed actions. In general, there is a greater tendency for proposed
solutions to be economically based among those who do not advocate the
rejection of prevailing development models.

The four agendas which focus on the ethical aspects of environment and
development generally agree that the pursuit of sustainability requires an
appropriate ethical framework and that living sustainably will mean moving
away from current values and belief systems which perpetuate social inequity
and environmental degradation.

The *NGO Alternative Treaty* criticizes the current development model
'founded on economic relations that bestow privilege on the market while
abusing nature and human beings – treating them as resources and sources of
income'. *Agenda Ya Wananchi* speaks out against 'a global lifestyle and value
system in which there is never enough and there is such a lot that is unnecessary'. The *Women's Action Agenda 21* blasts 'the current moral and ethical
double standards' that govern environment and development activities,

women's participation and social justice throughout the world. And *Caring for the Earth* warns that we must 'discourage those [values and ethics] that are incompatible with a sustainable way of life'.

Five years later

During the Earth Summit there was an attempt to draft an Earth Charter containing values to guide sustainability. It was not possible to reach an agreement in 1992, and the *Rio Declaration on Environment and Development* took the place of a separate charter. The task was taken up again by Green Cross and the Earth Council in 1995 in The Hague. After nearly two years of consultations, a Benchmark Draft Earth Charter has emerged. More consultations are planned and the quest continues for a widely accepted Earth Charter.

Health

Agenda 21	chapter 6: Protection and Promotion of Human Health
ASCEND 21	chapter 5: Health
Caring for the Earth	chapter 3: Improving the Quality of Human Life
Women's Action Agenda 21	Woman's Rights, Population Policies and Health
Voice of the Eagle	The Medicines

All agendas addressing health issues identify a need to improve the quality of human health. *ASCEND 21* says the most urgent requirement is to help the under-privileged, who are bearing the brunt of environmental health problems. The *Women's Action Agenda 21* points to the need to change top-down, demographically driven population policies and programmes which are eroding or preventing adequate health care.

The most common reason for poor human health is environmental degradation. *Agenda 21* cites insufficient and inappropriate development resulting in either poverty or over-consumption and an expanding world population. *Voice of the Eagle* specifies the current imbalance between the spiritual, emotional and physical aspects of lifestyle.

Major points of comparison among the agendas

ASCEND 21 and *Agenda 21* agree on the nature and cause of major human health problems and also on many general areas of suggested activity, including control of disease, urban health, measures for improving and protecting the health of the very poor and the need for preventive programmes. *Agenda 21* identifies specific activities, such as eliminating guinea-worm disease and eradicating polio by the year 2000.

Agenda 21 focuses on illness and problems of poor health, while *Caring for the Earth* discusses health as a quality-of-life issue. The underlying cause of health problems is interpreted very differently in the two documents. *Agenda 21* names over-consumption and inappropriate development models, while *Caring for the Earth* cites the lack of adequate investment in national social programmes. *Agenda 21* provides a much more detailed examination of activities to deal with poor health, while *Caring for the Earth* merely lists targets set by the WHO, such as a 50 per cent reduction in moderate malnutrition.

Agenda 21 and the *Women's Action Agenda 21* both link poor health with environmental degradation and over-consumption but they part company on the issue of population. *Agenda 21* primarily sees population growth placing stress on the carrying capacity of the Earth, while the *Women's Action Agenda 21* speaks out against 'demographically driven' population policies and programmes. Both documents emphasize the importance of improving the status of women, with the *Women's Action Agenda 21* encouraging the development of 'women-centred, women-managed reproductive health care and family planning'. *Agenda 21* avoids the family planning issue.

Both *Agenda 21* and *Voice of the Eagle* state that human health is deteriorating although *Voice of the Eagle* says this applies to spiritual and emotional as well as physical health. Naturally, different solutions are suggested. *Voice of the Eagle* focuses on holistic treatment and the recognition of 'natural medicines' as valuable and sacred, while *Agenda 21* emphasizes preventive practices.

In *Agenda 21*, indigenous peoples are singled out as a 'vulnerable group' with respect to health because 'their relationship with traditional lands has been fundamentally changed'. Suggested remedial activities include 'strengthening, through resources and self-management, preventative and curative health services' for indigenous peoples and their communities, and integrating traditional knowledge and experience into health systems. While this is not at odds with *Voice of the Eagle*, it is pointed out in the section called 'The Medicines' that pharmaceutical companies are profiting from the exploitation of the knowledge of indigenous medicine people. This point is not made in *Agenda 21*.

Five years later

Three research reports that look at the link between environment and health in 1997 conclude that not enough is being done to assess and address the health impacts of environmental change. An international study to measure public perceptions of the links between the environment and health found that a majority of people in all but one of the seventeen countries studied believe that environmental problems now affect their health.[32] A report from the International Institute of Concern for Public Health[33] urges creation of an International Environment Agency responsible for determining acceptable standards for protecting human health and the environment. An Environment

Canada report on the health implications of environmental change recommends that where there are threats of serious or irreversible damage to health, lack of full scientific certainty should be a reason to postpone cost-effective preventive measures. UNGASS stresses that health issues still need to be 'fully integrated into national and sub-national sustainable development plans and should be incorporated into project and programme development as a component of environmental impact assessments'.

These conclusions echo suggestions made in the 1992 agendas and demonstrate that many things remain the same five years after the Earth Summit.

Indigenous peoples

Agenda 21	chapter 26: Recognising and Strengthening the Role of Indigenous People and their Communities
NGO Alternative Treaties	International Treaty between Non-Governmental Organizations and Indigenous Peoples
Agenda Ya Wananchi	Appeal to Governments: Acknowledge Aboriginal Indigenous Land Rights

Three different perspectives emerge in the four documents which focus on indigenous peoples. *Agenda 21* examines the role that indigenous peoples can play in sustainable development, recognizing that their participation has been 'limited as a result of economic, social and historical factors'. *Agenda Ya Wananchi* and the International Treaty between Non-Governmental Organizations and Indigenous Peoples stress that denying the rights of indigenous peoples, including the right to self-determination or the rights to ownership of their lands, is causing destruction of the environment and of indigenous cultures. *Voice of the Eagle* is essentially spiritual guidance for achieving a more harmonious world. The *NGO Alternative Treaty* concerning indigenous peoples is different from the other alternative treaties in that it forms an agreement between the NGOs and another party.

In common with other communities called 'major groups' in *Agenda 21* (for example, women, business, science), the chapters in which indigenous peoples are highlighted as a topic include suggestions for actions and activities originating from both inside and outside the community. This has caused concern for indigenous peoples, who question the ability of others to speak on their behalf. This is one of the reasons why the *NGO Alternative Treaty* is an agreement with indigenous peoples rather than a set of statements on relevant issues by NGOs.

Agenda 21 differs from the two NGO documents by making no reference to the 'inalienable rights' of indigenous peoples to their land and to self-determination which are fundamental principles in the NGO agreement and in *Agenda Ya Wananchi*.

Major points of comparison among the agendas

Agenda 21 and the International Treaty between Non-Governmental Organizations and Indigenous Peoples illustrate a recognition of the immense contribution that indigenous peoples and their communities and knowledge base can make in helping to achieve a more environmentally sound future. Both observe that this can only happen if indigenous peoples are given the opportunity for genuine input into decision-making and if their cultures are not under constant threat of destruction.

The broad issue of enabling indigenous peoples to achieve sustainable development is central to this chapter of *Agenda 21*, while *Agenda Ya Wananchi* focuses specifically on the need for governments to recognize indigenous peoples' rights to self-determination and rightful ownership of pre-colonization lands. Among the actions proposed by *Agenda 21* is the enforcement of the ILO Indigenous and Tribal Peoples Convention which echoes the call for self-determination, although explicit mention of this is missing from *Agenda 21*.

Five years later

The role of stakeholders, including indigenous people, has been called 'one of the real successes of *Agenda 21*'.[34] The UNGASS review pointed out that 'the special needs, culture, traditions and expertise of indigenous people must be recognised', which is similar to what was recommended in *Agenda 21*.

Institutions

Agenda 21	chapter 38: International Institutional Arrangements
Agenda Ya Wananchi	Appeal to Governments: Democratise International Lending Institutions
ASCEND 21	chapter 16: Institutional Arrangements
Youth Action Guide	chapter 14: Development and Institutional Structure

These four agendas all take different approaches to institutions as an environment and development issue. *Agenda 21* looks at the need for international institutional arrangements to implement *Agenda 21*, with the emphasis on UN organizations. *ASCEND 21* takes a global approach to the institutional arrangements required to halt and reverse environmental degradation, including 'increased democratisation of institutes and decentralisation of decision-making in Eastern Europe and much of the Third World'. This focus on changes needed in Eastern Europe and the Third World is at odds with *Agenda Ya Wananchi*, which stresses changes in Northern institutions and governments.

Agenda Ya Wananchi and the *Youth Action Guide* make a case for changes in existing international institutions such as 'changes in social, economic and political institutions to allow social and economic development' (*Youth Action Guide*) and increased participation in decision-making in international lending institutions (*Agenda Ya Wananchi*). There is general agreement across the four agendas that international institutions play an important role in determining the socio-economic backdrop against which sustainable development can be pursued.

Major points of comparison among the agendas

Agenda 21 speaks to the institutional arrangements of UN agencies, including efforts aimed at 'revitalising the UN', to support the implementation of *Agenda 21*, while *Agenda Ya Wananchi* highlights international lending institutions with a call for more public participation in decisions on international financing.

The *Youth Action Guide* examines the institutional changes needed to enhance social and economic development. The youth agenda makes some general comments about the desired characteristics of international institutions, such as social accountability and social and geographical decentralization, that are not found in *Agenda 21*.

Five years later

The Commission on Sustainable Development (CSD) was set up in the aftermath of the Earth Summit to follow up on the implementation of *Agenda 21*. In some circles this caused confusion regarding UNEP's role in supporting sustainability.[35] UNDP was another UN agency which assumed major responsibility for overseeing *Agenda 21*. In particular, UNDP's Capacity 21 programme has helped a number of developing countries put together national sustainable development plans.

The UNGASS review clearly stated that

> the role of UNEP, as the principal United Nations body *in the field of the environment*, should be further enhanced [and] . . . UNDP should continue to strengthen its contribution to and programmes in sustainable development and the implementation of *Agenda 21* at all levels particularly in the area of promoting capacity-building (including through its Capacity 21 programme).

While this delineation of responsibilities clarifies the roles of these institutions, it does not really recognize the fundamental need to integrate environment and development objectives for sustainability to be achieved.

Local initiatives

Agenda 21   chapter 28: Local Authorities' Initiatives in Support
                     of *Agenda 21*
Caring for the Earth chapter 7: Enabling Communities to Care for their
                     own Environment

Although only two of the documents considered here give chapter-level status to local initiatives, virtually all of the agendas suggest and encourage activities at the community or local level to achieve more sustainable lifestyles.

Between *Agenda 21* and *Caring for the Earth*, *Agenda 21* focuses more specifically on using local government for local applications of *Agenda 21*. *Caring for the Earth* stresses making sustainable living a priority at the community level, although even stronger emphasis is given to individual commitments to lifestyle changes.

Major points of comparison between the agendas

Agenda 21 focuses specifically on its local application through local government, while *Caring for the Earth* presents a similar view of making sustainable living a priority at the community level without the emphasis on local government. Both documents recognize the importance of local participation and initiatives. In *Agenda 21* this is presented as part of multilevel government involvement in implementation of *Agenda 21* (for example, local, regional, national), while *Caring for the Earth* sees the priority as enabling communities to care for their own environment. *Caring for the Earth* and *Agenda 21* both suggest activities for improving local government planning and policy implementation with respect to input from individuals at the grassroots level. *Agenda 21* emphasizes international co-operation and dialogue between local authorities, while in *Caring for the Earth* the international element is in the form of proposed assistance for community environmental actions.

Five years later

During the 1997 review of progress it became apparent that the *Local Agendas 21* initiative has been among the most successful of all the recommendations that came forward during the Earth Summit. This is due in large part to the importance that local communities place on sustainability goals and to the significant efforts of the International Council for Local Environment Initiatives (ICLEI), headed by the dynamic Jeb Brugmann.

According to ICLEI,[36] following UNCED local government, national and international local government authorities, international bodies and UN agencies entered a period of experimentation with the implementation of the *Local Agenda 21* concept. The accumulation and exchange of practical experiences helped to identify a set of universal elements and factors for the success of *Local Agenda 21* planning.

> Since 1991, more than 1,800 local governments in 64 countries have established *Local Agenda 21* planning processes to engage their communities in *Agenda 21* implementation at the local level. Local governments and their communities have voluntarily assumed new responsibilities for global environmental problems, such as climate change, forest destruction and pollution of the seas.

Military

NGO Alternative Treaties	Treaty on Militarism, the Environment and Development
Agenda Ya Wananchi	Appeal to Governments: Reduce Military Spending by at Least Half
Youth '92	Peace

The three agendas which focus on military activities all advocate new definitions of security, including taking into account sustainability and the environment (*Agenda Ya Wananchi*), recognizing that 'peace is more than just the absence of war' (*Youth '92*) and acknowledging the 'links between militarism, debt, environmental degradation and maldevelopment' (*NGO Alternative Treaties*). All the agendas also strongly advocate reducing military spending in favour of alleviating poverty by providing for basic human needs. In addition, they call for diverting money spent for military purposes to control or repair environmental damage, a proposal commonly referred to as 'the peace dividend'. Although *Agenda 21* does not contain a chapter on peace or militarism, two of the principles in the Rio Declaration do, in part, echo the sentiments expressed above, including Principle 25 ('peace, development and environmental protection are interdependent and indivisible') and Principle 26 ('states shall resolve all their environmental disputes peacefully by appropriate means in accordance with the Charter of the United Nations').

The *Youth '92* document presents the most comprehensive background and the largest number of ideas for achieving peace, including security of the social and physical environment, harmony within and between individuals and with nature, and personal and spiritual peace.

Five years later

Militarism was again overlooked in the five-year follow-up activities. For some[37] this reflects a lack of recognition at the Earth Summit and in the succeeding years 'of the underlying cause of today's crisis – the unsustainable economic models that most of the world is currently following'. This includes the belief that 'free trade, multinational transnational corporations and militarism – some of the biggest contributors to today's crisis – were deliberately left off the agenda'. This point is dealt with more fully in Chapter 8.

NGOs

Agenda 21	chapter 27: Strengthening the Role of Non-Governmental Organisations: Partners for Sustainable Development
NGO Alternative Treaties	Treaty for NGO Co-operation and Sharing of Resources, Code of Conduct for NGOs, Communication, Information, Media and Networking

The role of non-governmental organizations in achieving a more sustainable future is not dealt with expressly in many of the documents compared here. However, the fact that all the agendas, with the exception of *Agenda 21* (which includes input from NGOs) were prepared by NGOs illustrates the importance these groups place on the work they are doing.

The strict definition of the term 'non-governmental organization' is just what it says: an organization which is not representative of a government. In recent years, there has been much debate about what qualifies as a 'non-governmental organization', particularly when provisions are made for NGO representation on advisory committees, commissions or UN delegations. In the area of environment and development, groups traditionally taking a more activist role in working for change have been considered to be NGOs. They include women's groups, youth groups, community groups and national and international groups formed to fight for specific issues such as saving old-growth forest.

Increasingly, a distinction is now being made between large, well-funded, international environment and development lobby groups such as WWF, Greenpeace or the Third World Network and small, locally based groups working on issues that directly affect them from a social, economic, environmental or spiritual perspective. These groups are more commonly known as grassroots organizations although they are still defined as NGOs under a variety of circumstances. Indigenous peoples often do not want to be seen as NGOs since they consider themselves to be nations. They are usually denied that status during, for instance, certain UN negotiations and therefore are sometimes found among the ranks of NGOs.

Groups which governments might consider to be NGOs such as scientific organizations or business and industry groups, often are not accepted as NGOs by non-governmental organizations working to build the political will for changes such as an alternative world economy based on fair trade rather than free trade. Scientific organizations have generally seen themselves as unbiased

41

providers of information rather than activists and therefore are not necessarily seen as working to change the *status quo*. Business and industrial organisations often do not enjoy the support of non-governmental activist organizations since, to many, they contributed to the current global environmental crisis.

Major points of comparison between the agendas

Although the *Treaty for NGO Co-operation and Sharing of Resources*, *Code of Conduct* and the *Code of Conduct for NGOs* are primarily documents aimed at the structure and ethics of NGO behaviour rather than issues of environment and development, they do correspond roughly with chapter 27 in *Agenda 21*. In areas where issues overlap, there is generally agreement between *Agenda 21* and the NGO documents (for instance, increase the participation of NGOs in decision-making).

Five years later

Five years after the Earth Summit it appears that the primary role of NGOs has shifted from one of identifying areas of controversy between the national governments and other actors for sustainability to more diagnostic activities. There is also greater evidence that the international politically sophisticated NGOs that participated in the UNCED process are now more fully involved in policy dialogue with other major actors, including business and government.[38]

Population

Agenda 21	chapter 5: Demographic Dynamics and Sustainability
NGO Alternative Treaties	Treaty on Population, Environment and Development
ASCEND 21	chapter 1: Population and Natural Resource Use
Caring for the Earth	chapter 5: Keeping within the Earth's Carrying Capacity
Women's Action Agenda 21	Women's Rights, Population Policies and Health
Youth Action Guide	chapter 2: Population
Changing Course	chapter 10: Leadership for Sustainable Development in Developing Countries

The population issue is delicate because of its ties with culture and religion. This was underlined by the tension surrounding the United Nations Conference on Population and Development held in Cairo in 1994 following threats from groups demanding that discussion on sensitive issues such as birth control or abortion be limited or banned. The reasons given in various agendas for the existence of population problems illustrate the variety of views in this area.

The seven agendas which address population display a range of perspectives, some more straightforward than others. The *Youth Action Guide* focuses on high population growth as the most pressing problem; other agendas emphasize the link between the size of the Earth's population and degradation of natural resources through pressure on carrying capacity (*Agenda 21, ASCEND 21, Caring for the Earth*). Several agendas consider the need for changes in population policies and programmes. The *NGO Alternative Treaty on Population, Environment and Development* says that the international community must address problems arising from the relationship between population and environment and unequal consumption patterns and access to resources. The *Women's Action Agenda 21* criticizes 'top-down, demographically driven population policies and programmes' as being at the heart of environmental degradation. *Changing Course* frames the problem in terms of the increasing difficulty of meeting the basic needs of a growing population.

The *NGO Alternative Treaty* skirts the issue of controlling population growth and instead focuses on militarism, debt, structural adjustment and trade policies which the signatories feel are being promoted by corporations and international financial and trade institutions and are causing environmental degradation. *Agenda 21, ASCEND 21* and *Caring for the Earth* all point to unsustainable consumption patterns as perpetuating the difficulties in meeting the needs of a growing population. Only *Caring for the Earth* directly states that the rate of population growth is a problem. Other agendas focus on the poor status of women, erroneously blaming women's fertility rates (*Women's Action Agenda 21*) and limited access to and negative attitudes towards family planning (*Youth '92*). *Youth '92* also points out that the lack of social welfare programmes encourages people to have children as security in old age and that high infant mortality rates can also lead to large families.

Major points of comparison among the agendas

Agenda 21 does not set out the reasons for the link between demographic and environmental problems as clearly as the *NGO Alternative Treaties* but examples of measures proposed to alleviate the problems indicate some common ground (for example, improving the status of women). *Agenda 21* gives more precise examples of proposed activities (such as modelling of migration flows due to climate change).

The overall problem and the conditions leading to its existence are explained in essentially the same manner in *Agenda 21* and *ASCEND 21*. Many of the same activities are proposed, although *ASCEND 21* puts greater emphasis on research into such issues as 'the question of limits to carrying capacity of the Earth System for a human population'. Improving the status of women is only mentioned once in chapter 1 of *ASCEND 21*, while it is a recurrent theme in chapter 5 of *Agenda 21*.

The carrying capacity of the Earth with respect to population continues to be a contentious issue. This can be seen in the different language of *Caring for the Earth* and *Agenda 21*. *Caring for the Earth* bluntly states the concern that the human population will exceed the Earth's carrying capacity. *Agenda 21* speaks of 'placing stress' on the Earth's carrying capacity. This difference can also be seen in the reasons given for the problem. *Caring for the Earth* simply says that it is population growth. *Agenda 21*, while recognizing the problem of a growing world population, points also to unsustainable production. Proposed activities also reflect this difference in emphasis. Both chapters propose programmes to improve health care and the status of women, although only *Caring for the Earth* mentions family planning services.

Agenda 21 and the *Youth Action Guide* adopt a similar definition of the population question: both agree on the need to improve reproductive health care and work to improve the status of women. The main difference is that *Agenda 21* focuses on demographics (such as migration) while the *Youth Action Guide* stresses the need for improved access to family planning and for more open discussion. Family planning is not raised in *Agenda 21* and neither are the specific recommendations for preventing the spread of AIDS (for instance, advertising campaigns for men to use condoms) proposed by the *Youth Action Guide*.

Changing Course focuses on the gap between access to basic human needs and the number of people on the planet and is forthright about the need to lower population growth, an issue which *Agenda 21* studiously avoids. Both documents emphasize the need to improve the status of women. *Changing Course* advocates increased availability of contraceptives, which is not found in *Agenda 21*.

Five years later

The rate of population growth has decreased slightly in the years since the Earth Summit. According to Worldwatch Institute,[39]

> While the overall number of people continues to increase, the annual rate of growth has been slowly dropping from its record high in 1963 . . . the significance of this decline is limited, however, due to the expanding base population: the 2.2 per-cent growth rate in 1963 yielded 69 million more people, but the 1.4 per-cent growth rate in 1996 produced an additional 80 million.

Urbanization

Agenda 21	chapter 7: Promoting Sustainable Human Settlement Development
NGO Alternative Treaties	Treaty on Urbanization

Agenda Ya Wananchi	NGO Commitment 9: Rebuilding of Cities in Balance with Nature/Appeal to Governments: Rebuild Cities in Balance with Nature
Caring for the Earth	chapter 12: Human Settlements
Youth Action Guide	chapter 5: Urbanization

The five agendas with chapters on human settlements and urbanization agree that living conditions within cities are deteriorating. Growing numbers of city dwellers are unable to meet their basic needs for food, fresh water and shelter, and environmental degradation is getting worse. *Agenda Ya Wananchi* states simply that 'cities are not in balance with nature'. *Agenda 21* blames the fate of the urban poor on 'low levels of investment in the urban sector attributable to the overall resource constraints in certain countries'. *Caring for the Earth* cites the failure of local and national governments. The *Youth Action Guide* points to a lack of investment in rural areas, forcing people to move to the city to find work, and also indicates that social conditions are poor due to a lack of a sense of community and decentralized decision-making. The *NGO Alternative Treaty on Urbanization* cites 'unlimited greed' fuelling the disparity between rich and poor, and industrial growth 'based on expansion and consumption' which has contributed to the displacement of rural inhabitants.

Major points of comparison among the agendas

The documents have a common starting point with broad agreement on the definition of the problems and the reasons for their existence. In general, *Agenda 21* gives more concrete suggestions for action taking into account land-use planning, provision of environmental infrastructure, water, sanitation and solid-waste management.

There is a slightly different interpretation of the nature of the problem. *Agenda 21* focuses on the deterioration of existing cities resulting from 'resource constraints'. *Agenda Ya Wananchi* says that cities are becoming unpleasant places in which to live because they are not built in balance with the natural environment. Suggested activities for alleviating the problem reflect the difference in perspective on human settlements between the two documents. *Agenda 21* encourages governments to find the resources to improve current living conditions in cities using foreign aid if necessary, while *Agenda Ya Wananchi* calls for urban planning and development based on ecological principles.

Caring for the Earth also draws attention to the problem of expanding urbanization. The reason for deteriorating conditions in the cities, according to *Caring for the Earth*, is the failure of local and national governments. *Agenda 21* refers to a more vague 'low level of investment in the urban sector', placing particular emphasis on the belief that this is more prevalent in some countries than others. Both *Caring for the Earth* and *Agenda 21* propose improving urban infrastructure. *Caring for the Earth* looks to local government for solutions based on long-range ecosystem-based planning, while *Agenda 21* advises the use of modern planning methods and tools at the national level and raises the question of assistance for poorer countries in order to achieve sustainable human settlement goals.

The problems surrounding urban settlements are defined in a similar manner in *Agenda 21* and the *Youth Action Guide* (for example, urban homelessness, lack of access to clean water, unemployment). The *Youth Action Guide* places slightly greater emphasis on the need to stop the growth of urbanization through measures such as improving small farmers' access to credit and their rights to land ownership, in addition to improving existing conditions in urban areas.

Women

Agenda 21	chapter 24: Global Action for Women towards Sustainable and Equitable Development
NGO Alternative Treaties	A Global Women's Treaty for NGOs Seeking a Just and Healthy Planet
Agenda Ya Wananchi	NGO Commitment 7: Ensure Women's Equal and Integral Participation in Decision-making, Appeal to Governments: Ratify and Implement Women's Rights Legislation
Women's Action Agenda 21	The entire agenda
Global Assembly of Women	Role of Women in the Environment

The subject of women is raised, in one form or another, in all the eleven agendas referred to in this study. Although the *Women's Action Agenda 21* was developed solely by women, it does not isolate women as a topic. In the preamble to the *Women's Action Agenda 21* an appeal is made 'to all women and men to join in this call for profound and immediate transformation in human values and activities'. Issues singled out for action by the *Women's Action Agenda 21* include democratic rights, diversity and solidarity; a code of environmental ethics and accountability; women, militarism and the environment; foreign debt and trade; women, poverty, land rights, food security and credit; women's rights, population policies and health; biodiversity and biotechnology; nuclear power and alternative energy; science and technology transfer; women's consumer power; and information and education.

Five agendas, however, do address women and their role in sustainable development as a separate priority area. *Agenda 21*, *A Global Women's Treaty for NGOs Seeking a Just and Healthy Planet*, *Agenda Ya Wananchi* and the *Global Assembly of Women* identify the exclusion or under-involvement of women in decision-making and positions of leadership as a major problem. *Voice of the Eagle* stresses the need for women to be respected.

Major points of comparison among the agendas

There is a good deal of agreement among the agendas particularly with respect to problem definition and the direction of proposed actions. The NGO document goes further than *Agenda 21* in linking the inadequate representation of women in many areas to broader problems such as militarism and a general lack of respect for cultural diversity.

The *NGO Alternative Treaty* and *Agenda 21* emphasize the unequal partici-pation of women in policy- and decision-making and *Agenda 21* identifies this as a factor with the potential to undermine the successful implementation of *Agenda 21*. There is a shared recognition of the need to increase the number of women in decision-making roles and on the importance of implementing the Nairobi Forward-looking Strategies for the Advancement of Women. *Agenda 21* advocates the use of planning tools such as environmental impact assess-ment and gender impact assessment, while *Agenda Ya Wananchi* underlines the commitment of NGOs to fight for the changes necessary to achieve equality for women.

The *Global Assembly of Women* asserts that the proportion and number of women holding senior positions should be increased.

While *Agenda 21* goes into greater detail than *Voice of the Eagle*, the basic premise is the same: women must be respected. In *Voice of the Eagle* this is because they are, like Mother Earth, 'sacred givers of life'. In *Agenda 21* it is because they are necessary for implementing *Agenda 21*.

In the years since the Earth Summit a number of international gatherings that have relevance for women have taken place. These include the International Conference on Population and Development (ICPD) held in Cairo in 1994 and the World Summit for Social Development held in Copenhagen in 1995. But according to the Women's Environment and Development Organization,[40] 'the Platform for Action adopted by the UN Fourth World Conference on Women, held in Beijing in September 1995, is the strongest statement of international consensus on women's equality and empowerment that has ever been agreed upon by governments'. WEDO's conclusions, supported by the examples in chapter 7, indicate that progress has indeed occurred in the parts of *Agenda 21* relevant to women and, in a number of cases, in the *Women's Action Agenda 21*. WEDO believes that five years after the Earth Summit the imperatives of the global economy seem to be outrun-ning the post-Rio agenda and national budget allocations are not sufficiently in tune with post-Rio needs. Neither are national policies that seek and main-tain foreign capital investment.

5

THE WELL-BEING OF ECOSYSTEMS

An ecosystem is a unit that includes a dynamic complex of plants, animals and their physical environment that interact in many ways. Its management implies a holistic approach incorporating such well-known concepts as multiple uses and purposes, future trends as well as social and economic values and the desirable long-term objectives implied in sustainability.[41] In this chapter, components of sustainability most closely related to ecosystem management and degradation are explored. Table 5.1 provides a summary of the agendas that focus on ecological issues.

Agriculture

Agenda 21	chapter 14: Promoting Sustainable Agriculture and Rural Development
NGO Alternative Treaties	Food Security Treaty, Sustainable Agriculture Treaty
Agenda Ya Wananchi	Appeal to Governments: Promote Sustainable Agriculture
ASCEND 21	chapter 2: Agriculture, Land Use and Degradation
Caring for the Earth	chapter 13: Farm and Range Lands
Youth Action Guide	chapter 4: Food Production and Consumption Patterns
Changing Course	chapter 9: Sustainable Management of Renewable Resources: Agriculture and Forestry

The availability of food (food security) and the way in which it is produced (agricultural practices) are the recurrent themes in the seven agendas which make agriculture a priority issue. Food security is examined in terms of the quantity of food (*Agenda 21*) and distribution (*NGO Alternative Treaty*, the *Youth Action Guide*).

The agendas agree that most farming methods are unsustainable in the long run, but they differ dramatically on the reasons for current environment-

Table 5.1 Ecological issues covered in the agendas

	Agriculture	Atmosphere	Biodiversity	Biotechnology	Deforestation	Desertification	Energy	Land resources	Marine environment	Nuclear issues	Science	Technology	Waste management	Water
Agenda 21	✓	✓	✓	✓	✓	✓	✗	✓	✓	✓	✓	✓	✓	✓
NGO Alternative Treaties	✓	✓	✓	✓	✓	✓	✗	✗	✓	✓	✗	✓	✓	✓
Agenda Ya Wananchi	✓	✓	✓	✓	✗	✗	✗	✗	✗	✓	✗	✓	✗	✗
ASCEND 21	✓	✓	✓	✗	✗	✗	✗	✗	✗	✓	✓	✓	✓	✓
Caring for the Earth	✗	✓	✓	✓	✓	✗	✓	✗	✓	✗	✗	✗	✗	✓
Women's Action Agenda 21	✗	✗	✓	✓	✗	✗	✓	✗	✗	✗	✓	✓	✗	✓
Global Assembly of Women and the Environment	✗	✗	✗	✗	✗	✗	✓	✗	✗	✓	✗	✓	✓	✗
Youth '92	✓	✗	✓	✓	✗	✓	✗	✓	✗	✗	✗	✗	✗	✓
Youth Action Guide	✓	✓	✗	✗	✗	✗	✓	✗	✗	✗	✗	✗	✓	✓
Voice of the Eagle	✗	✓	✗	✗	✓	✗	✗	✗	✗	✗	✗	✗	✓	✗
Changing Course	✓	✗	✓	✗	✓	✗	✓	✗	✗	✗	✗	✓	✗	✓

✓ = a major priority area ✗ = not a major area

and development-related agricultural problems. *Agenda 21* and *ASCEND 21* blame poor land management. *Changing Course* criticizes agricultural markets for being neither as open nor as competitive as they should be. *Caring for the Earth* and the *Youth Action Guide* are concerned that not enough food is being produced to meet local needs while farmers concentrate on cash crops for export. The *NGO Alternative Treaties* on food security and sustainable agriculture blame a dominant global socio-economic and political system which promotes industrial agricultural production.

Major points of comparison among the agendas

The *NGO Alternative Treaty* says that political problems cause poor food distribution and hunger, and *Agenda 21* maintains that simply increasing the quantity of food will alleviate hunger and starvation. These different perspectives are reflected in the solutions recommended by the two agendas, although both documents stress the need to adopt more sustainable models of agricultural production.

Agenda Ya Wananchi also gives prominence to sustainable agriculture, and its proposed actions are similar to those in *Agenda 21*, including reducing reliance on pesticides in favour of organic farming practices.

Agenda 21 highlights a growing population's increasing demand for food, while *ASCEND 21* identifies the main problem as the ever-increasing demand for land coupled with the worsening conditions on available lands such as pests, disease and drought. There is agreement that the problem is caused by under-use or mismanagement of high-potential land. *ASCEND 21*'s proposals focus on enhancing land productivity while decreasing degradation by applying technologies such as 'the global benefits of the biotechnology option' [p. 87]. While biotechnology is discussed in *Agenda 21* (chapter 16), it is not raised in chapter 14. *Agenda 21* is more concerned with the social aspects of sustainable agriculture such as the need for improved access to quality agricultural lands for women and for broader participation in agricultural decisions.

Agenda 21 says that many people are not getting enough to eat because of inefficient and undesirable land use. *Caring for the Earth* blames poverty and the failure to give priority to local food production to meet local needs. Many of the proposed activities are the same and include soil conservation and enhancing soil fertility. *Caring for the Earth* gives greater recognition to the importance of integrating the numerous systems, including crop, livestock, water and soil systems.

The *Youth Action Guide* discusses food distribution and food shortage, pointing to economic instruments such as inappropriate subsidies as well as excessive consumption of meat and the production of cash crops instead of food to meet local demands. The *Youth Action Guide* suggests measures such as small farming co-operatives and reduced meat consumption.

Agenda 21 and *Changing Course* take slightly different approaches to farming, with *Agenda 21* concentrating on increasing food security and *Changing Course* focusing on unsustainable farming and marketing practices. Both documents advocate forest conservation and policies that recognize the multiple roles of forests as well as more widespread use of sustainable farming practices, including integrated pest management. *Changing Course* advocates eliminating agricultural subsidies, a suggestion that is not found in *Agenda 21*. Forestry and agriculture are covered in separate chapters of *Agenda 21*, although the links between them are recognized (for example, 'analyse and identify possibilities for economic integration of agricultural and forest activities'). *Changing Course* discusses them together.

Five years later

Despite continued gains in food production, people in many parts of the world remain hungry and malnourished, and, with global population growing by 90 million a year, demand for food will intensify. Meanwhile, unsustainable agricultural practices are compromising the natural resource base upon which all food production depends. In many regions land productivity has begun to stagnate or decline. Science and technology offer some solutions but, without significant policy changes and initiatives, scientists can have only a limited impact.

Atmosphere

Agenda 21	chapter 9: Protection of the Atmosphere
NGO Alternative Treaties	Alternative Non-Governmental Agreement on Climate Change, Treaty on Energy
Agenda Ya Wananchi	Appeal to Governments: Reduce Greenhouse Gas Emissions
ASCEND 21	chapter 7: Atmosphere and Climate/chapter 4: Energy
Caring for the Earth	chapter 4: Conserving the Earth's Vitality and Diversity
Youth '92	Protection of Natural Resources: Biodiversity/Forests/Biotechnology
Youth Action Guide	chapter 6: The Greenhouse Effect/chapter 7: Ozone Depletion and Acid Rain

Solutions to global atmospheric problems are often the very same measures needed to combat local and regional air pollution. On all fronts, the most important step that any nation can take is gradually to rely more on renewable, non-polluting sources of energy for power plants, industries and transportation, and to encourage more efficient use of all energy sources.

Seven agendas examine the atmosphere issue, all focusing on the effect of man-made pollutants including greenhouse gases (*NGO Alternative Treaties, Agenda Ya Wananchi,* the *Youth Action Guide*) and the resultant potential for or existence of global climate change (*ASCEND 21, Caring for the Earth, Youth '92*). Agendas agree about the need to halt depletion of stratospheric ozone (*Agenda 21, ASCEND 21, Caring for the Earth, Agenda Ya Wananchi,* the *Youth Action Guide*), a problem that is responding well to actions initiated under the *Montreal Protocol on Substances that Deplete the Ozone Layer.*

Caring for the Earth and the two youth agendas all express concern about acid rain, while *Agenda 21* and *ASCEND 21* both identify the need for improved understanding of the effect of human activity on the environment. All the agendas which concern themselves with the atmosphere agree that current approaches to development and consumption are causing damage. Atmospheric deterioration is a result of human activities (*Caring for the Earth*) such as unsustainable energy use (*Agenda 21, NGO Alternative Treaties, Youth '92,* the *Youth Action Guide*) and powerful, non-accountable corporations causing social and environmental problems (*NGO Alternative Treaties*). Growing population and associated consumption and waste production are also cited as major factors (*ASCEND 21*) and both youth agendas draw attention to the harmful effects of deforestation and agriculture. *Youth '92* points out that atmospheric problems are principally the responsibility of industrialized countries, which produce most of the pollutants going into the air.

Major points of comparison among the agendas

There is an apparent consensus on the important atmospheric problems including climatic change and ozone depletion. The *NGO Alternative Treaties* articulate an underlying cause of the problem, while *Agenda 21* does not. Both groups point out the benefits of energy conservation and the use of alternative (including renewable) sources of energy. The *NGO Alternative Treaties* emphasize the need to work for change in this area. *Agenda Ya Wananchi* says it is the responsibility of governments of the North to implement the necessary changes.

Agenda 21 and *ASCEND 21* address the need for better understanding of atmospheric processes and for attention to urban air pollution, emissions from transport and industrial sources, acid rain, ozone depletion and global warming. *Agenda 21* does not offer a reason for these problems but *ASCEND 21* names growing consumption and production associated with a growing population as important underlying factors. Proposed remedial activities are similar, although *ASCEND 21* is more explicit in emphasizing the importance of scientific research in developing policies and programmes based on up-to-date data collection, analysis and modelling.

Agenda 21 puts slightly greater emphasis on improving understanding of the processes that influence atmospheric change, while *Caring for the Earth* is more direct in identifying global pollution and ecosystem destruction as the sources of atmospheric problems. Proposed activities in *Agenda 21* are broad, and fall, for the most part, within the realm of national governments. *Caring for the Earth* suggests some of the same activities but includes local measures to improve air quality and advocates lobbying and political campaigns for regulations and economic incentives to improve and protect the atmosphere.

While *Agenda 21* calls for improved understanding of the processes affecting the global atmosphere, *Youth '92* begins from the premise that climate change has already begun. *Youth '92*'s call for increased use of alternative energy sources such as solar and wind power finds support in *Agenda 21*. *Youth '92* blames the countries of the North for most of the damage to the atmosphere and demands that the North pay for the clean-up. This last point is not included in *Agenda 21*.

Agenda 21 and the *Youth Action Guide* agree that ozone depletion is a serious problem but, while the *Youth Action Guide* asserts that climate warming is a certainty, *Agenda 21* merely calls for improved understanding of atmospheric conditions. The *Youth Action Guide* gives several reasons why atmospheric quality is deteriorating (such as burning of fossil fuels, deforestation, landfill sites). *Agenda 21* does not directly address the question of cause. The *Youth Action Guide* and *Agenda 21* both propose the use of more energy-efficient technology, increased use of renewable fuels (*Youth Action Guide* goes further to suggest economic incentives to achieve this) and acceptance of the Montreal Protocol.

Five years later

As pointed out by UNGASS, 'despite the adoption of the [Climate Change] Convention, the emission and concentration of greenhouse gases (GHGs) continues to rise, even as scientific evidence assembled by the Intergovernmental Panel on Climate Change (IPCC) and other relevant bodies continues to diminish the uncertainties and points ever more strongly to the severe risk of global climate change'. According to Climate Network Europe,[42] the global economic recession led to slashed environment and energy budgets in areas critical to climate policy. For this reason, most countries will fail to achieve even the basic targets which they set for themselves (a stabilization of concentrations of GHGs in the atmosphere by the year 2000 using 1990 as a baseline). Some Scandinavian members of the European Union, such as Denmark and Sweden as well as the Netherlands, have taken a number of leading initiatives (for example, CO_2/energy taxes, minimum efficiency standards, support for energy efficiency, the co-generation of heat and electricity, and expanded use of renewable energy).

Biodiversity

Agenda 21	chapter 15: Conservation of Biological Diversity
NGO Alternative Treaties	Citizens' Commitment on Biodiversity, Draft Protocol on Scientific Research Components for the Conservation of Biodiversity, Marine Biodiversity Treaty
Agenda Ya Wananchi	Appeal to Governments: Compensation for Traditional Biological Knowledge
ASCEND 21	chapter 11: Biodiversity
Caring for the Earth	chapter 4: Conserving the Earth's Vitality and Diversity/chapter 13: Farm and Range Lands
Women's Action Agenda 21	Biodiversity and Biotechnology
Youth '92	Protection of Natural Resources: Biodiversity/Forests/Biotechnology
Voice of the Eagle	The Medicines

All the agendas listed above bemoan the current decline in biological diversity evidenced by an accelerating rate of extinction of plants, animals, fungi and micro-organisms both on land and in the sea. For some (*Agenda Ya Wananchi*, the *Women's Action Agenda 21*, *Youth '92*) the biodiversity issue is directly connected to biotechnology, and discussing one means discussing the other.[43] An example is the threat to natural biological diversity from genetically engineered organisms released into the environment (the *Women's Action Agenda 21*).

Various types of human activity are blamed for the biodiversity crisis, including powerful modern technology (*NGO Alternative Treaties*), population growth (*ASCEND 21*), loss of habitat through deforestation (*Youth '92*) and other activities (*ASCEND 21*, the *Women's Action Agenda 21*), the transfer of species from one region to another and its disruptive effect on ecosystems (*ASCEND 21*), exploitation of endangered species by hunters, poachers and tourists (*Youth '92*), and attempts by commercial interests from developed countries to control the natural heritage of the South (the *Women's Action Agenda 21*).

Major points of comparison among the agendas

The greatest difference between *Agenda 21* and the *NGO Alternative Treaties* lies in the priorities for action. Although there are similarities (such as inviting and enhancing the participation and support of local communities to preserve biodiversity), NGOs emphasize the need to change development patterns and practices on an international scale. *Agenda 21* promotes the view that whatever steps are taken, 'all states have the right to exploit their own biological resources pursuant to their environmental practices'.

In the biodiversity issue there is little common ground between *Agenda Ya Wananchi* and *Agenda 21*. *Agenda 21* identifies the general problem of a global decline in biodiversity. In contrast, *Agenda Ya Wananchi* homes in on issues not touched by *Agenda 21*, including preventing the patenting of life forms and genetic material.

ASCEND 21 pinpoints 'over-consumption by inhabitants of the industrialized nations as well as by relatively wealthy citizens of developing nations' as a major cause of species loss, while *Agenda 21* goes with the more general 'human activity'. The two documents, however, propose many of the same activities, including *in situ* conservation, increased training of specialists throughout the world and recognition of the importance of indigenous and local community knowledge. In *Agenda 21* this last point carries the proviso 'subject to national legislation'.

Caring for the Earth goes further than *Agenda 21* in saying that the rate of species decline is increasing and that evolutionary conditions are changing. The two documents propose many of the same activities (for example, participation of local communities in biodiversity preservation, *in situ* and *ex situ* protection of biological diversity and documentation of important areas of biodiversity). The issue of intellectual property rights is not raised in this chapter of *Agenda 21*, but *Caring for the Earth* states that intellectual property right regimes should not be an obstacle to farmers or other communities needing genetic material.

Agenda 21 treats biodiversity and biotechnology as separate issues, unlike the *Women's Action Agenda 21*. This highlights the documents' different perspectives on biotechnology, with *Agenda 21* seeing it as a possible solution for environmental problems and the *Women's Action Agenda 21* taking a much more cautious approach which emphasizes the risk to current biodiversity levels from genetically engineered organisms. The *Women's Action Agenda 21* sees a threat to developing countries from biotechnology companies in the North who are patenting life forms in the South in an attempt to control gene banks. This issue is not addressed in *Agenda 21*. Both agendas propose greater participation by local communities in protecting biodiversity and assessing the safety of biotechnology, but the *Women's Action Agenda 21* also proposes restrictions on biotechnology such as testing and releasing organisms only in the country of origin.

Agenda 21 and *Youth '92* agree that there is a global decline in biodiversity and that forests are being destroyed at an unsustainable rate. Both propose implementing sustainable forestry practices. Unlike *Agenda 21*, *Youth '92* links the issues of biodiversity and biotechnology. Both agendas see a role for local populations in decisions regarding biotechnology, but *Youth '92* advocates a ban on the patenting of genetically engineered organisms which *Agenda 21* does not mention. *Youth '92* also calls for strict regulation of all biotechnological activity, while *Agenda 21* focuses on the development and application of biotechnology.

Technical terms like 'biodiversity' are not found in *Voice of the Eagle*, primarily because it outlines spiritual beliefs. *Agenda 21* emphasizes the technical requirements for conserving biodiversity. In *Voice of the Eagle* the biodiversity issue is expressed through the importance of protecting, with respect, sacred plants used for medicines.

Five years later

The World Conservation Union (IUCN), a world leader in biodiversity issues, prepared a review of progress on the implementation of the *Convention on Biological Diversity* (CBD).[44] The CBD includes most of the recommendations made in the agendas discussed above. In their report IUCN observed that, 'because the *Convention on Biological Diversity* has been in force for only three years, it is still too early to measure its impact on biodiversity on the ground, or even to expect progress in the form of modified national policies. Even so, indications are that significant progress has been made on a number of fronts.'

Among the IUCN's findings are the following: 92 per cent of parties to the CBD say that they have increased access to information since the entry into force of the CBD; 65 per cent have used information provided through the CBD to develop their activities; 65 per cent are preparing a national biodiversity strategy or action plan (and 88 per cent have developed other strategies or plans related to biodiversity issues). At least partly in response to the CBD 78 per cent have identified important ecosystems and habitats; 58 per cent have strengthened measures for the conservation and sustainable use of these ecosystems and habitats since the ratification of the CBD; 58 per cent have developed and applied new approaches to sustainable forest management, most of which are at least partially taken in response to the CBD. And 70 per cent have carried out systematic inventories of wild biodiversity at the special level, most in response to the CBD.

Biotechnology

Agenda 21	chapter 16: Environmentally Sound Management of Biotechnology
NGO Alternative Treaties	Citizens' Commitments on Biotechnology
Agenda Ya Wananchi	Appeal to Governments: Compensation for Traditional Biological Knowledge
Caring for the Earth	chapter 4: Conserving the Earth's Vitality and Diversity/chapter 13: Farm and Range Lands
Women's Action Agenda 21	Biodiversity and Biotechnology
Youth '92	Protection of Natural Resources: Biodiversity/Forests/Biotechnology

In four out of the six agendas that make biotechnology a priority issue the subject is directly tied to biodiversity in the form of a threat to natural biological diversity from genetically engineered organisms (the *Women's Action Agenda 21*, *Youth '92*, *Caring for the Earth*) and species loss in the South because of the economic activities and interests of the North (*Agenda Ya Wananchi, Youth '92*). *Agenda 21* and the NGO *Alternative Treaty* – Citizens' Commitments on Biotechnology – both advocate an international agreement on principles which would guide work in the field of biotechnology 'to engender public trust and confidence, to promote the sustainable application of biotechnology and to establish appropriate enabling mechanisms, especially in developing countries' (*Agenda 21*), as well as to ensure 'respect for traditional knowledge and biotechnology research oriented towards the common good' (*NGO Alternative Treaties*). The need to establish mechanisms which recognize the contributions of traditional biological genetic material along with an appropriate compensation and royalties scheme is a theme found in *Agenda Ya Wananchi* and *Youth '92*.

Biotechnology is one of the most controversial issues raised in environment and development. For many, it is heavily laden with ethical dilemmas such as who gets access to biotechnology and whether an individual or corporation can own a life form just by patenting it. Exploitation of the resources of the South by interests from the North, in this case removing genetic material from the country of origin to be studied, duplicated and perhaps patented elsewhere, is another hotly contested issue.

Major points of comparison among the agendas

In general, *Agenda 21* concentrates on the potential benefits of biotechnology. The other documents emphasize the sensitive nature and possible dangers of biotechnology research along with the need for safety regulations and public involvement in decision-making. The *NGO Alternative Treaty* calls for a ban on the patenting of life forms, whereas *Agenda 21* does not mention patents. The *Women's Action Agenda 21* links biodiversity and biotechnology, emphasizing the risk posed to current levels of biodiversity from genetically released organisms.

Five years later

Biosafety as it relates to biotechnology remains a pressing issue. The UNGASS review emphasized this point by stating that it is necessary rapidly to complete 'the biosafety protocol under the convention on Biological Diversity, on the understanding that the UNEP International Technical Guidelines for Safety in Biotechnology may be used as an interim mechanism during its development, and to complement it after its conclusion'.

Deforestation

Agenda 21	chapter 11: Combating Deforestation
NGO Alternative Treaties	Forest Treaty, Treaty on Cerrados
Caring for the Earth	chapter 14: Forest Lands/chapter 4: Conserving the Earth's Vitality and Diversity
Youth Action Guide	chapter 8: Forest Management
Voice of the Eagle	The Trees
Changing Course	chapter 9: Sustainable Management of Renewable Resources: Agriculture and Forestry

The agendas posit a variety of reasons for the continuing rapid disappearance of the world's forests. These range from simple forestry mismanagement (*Changing Course*, *Caring for the Earth*, the *Youth Action Guide*, *NGO Alternative Treaties*) and bad trading practices (*NGO Alternative Treaties*, the *Youth Action Guide*) to a failure to recognize the unique role of trees (*Agenda 21*) in giving life and purifying the air (*Voice of the Eagle*). *Changing Course* blames a lack of open and competitive markets, *Caring for the Earth* says that many land-use practices are incompatible with forests, and the *Youth Action Guide* points the finger at international financial institutions which pressure countries to exploit forest resources in order to repay debts.

Major points of comparison among the agendas

The *NGO Alternative Treaties* include a list of pledges which overlap with most of the programme areas in the deforestation chapter of *Agenda 21*. The major difference is that the NGOs emphasize their commitment to action.

Both *Agenda 21* and *Caring for the Earth* see poor forest management as one of the principal reasons for deforestation. *Agenda 21* questions the adequacy of forest planning which tends to overlook the many roles – ecological, economic, social and cultural – played by forested lands. *Caring for the Earth* sees a need for more long-term planning.

While *Agenda 21* focuses on problems stemming from forests' multiple roles, the *Youth Action Guide* considers deforestation's side effects, such as flooding and desertification. Both documents see mismanagement of forests as the main reason for their decline, but the *Youth Action Guide* goes further, identifying a lack of political will to minimize deforestation and pressure from international financial institutions for countries to exploit forest resources for debt repayment. The focus of proposed activities is also slightly different, with *Agenda 21* suggesting general policies and programmes (enhancing forestry education, especially graduate and postgraduate degrees), while the *Youth Action Guide* makes more specific proposals such as including environmental studies in business management courses.

The multiple roles played by trees and forests are recognized in *Agenda 21* and *Voice of the Eagle*. Both documents urge forest conservation, although *Voice of the Eagle* suggests that trees should be cut only for ceremonial purposes, shelter and medicine. *Agenda 21* and *Changing Course* take the same line on managing forests, advocating conservation and forestry policies that recognize the multiple roles played by forests.

Five years later

The negotiation of the Forest Principles at UNCED has been described as 'torturous'[45] and, indeed, many of the negotiation sessions went on late into the night with the final session ending at four o'clock in the morning. From all that effort there is relatively little to report on in terms of progress in implementation. In the primarily NGO review of progress this outcome was perhaps predictable due to 'the failure to deal adequately with underlying causes of environmental degradation and the reluctance of Northern countries to take responsibility for their wasteful patterns of consumption'.[46]

The Intergovernmental Panel on Forests (IPF) is one initiative on forests that has emerged as a result of UNCED. It was set up in 1995 by the CBD and it is still too recent to gauge its impact. A number of the Forest Principles can be found among the recommendations in the Convention on Biological Diversity that has aided forward movement on the deforestation issue as outlined in *Agenda 21*.

Desertification

Agenda 21	chapter 12: Managing Fragile Ecosystems: Combating Desertification and Drought
NGO Alternative Treaties	Treaty Regarding Arid and Semi-arid Zones
Youth '92	Protection of Natural Resources: Land, Soil, Desertification

In *Agenda 21* and the *NGO Alternative Treaty Regarding Arid and Semi-arid Zones* the major desertification issue is defined as the degradation of arid and semi-arid lands. *Youth '92* defines the problem more broadly, linking poor land-use management, loss of soil fertility and deforestation with increasing desertification. *Agenda 21* blames climatic variations and the somewhat vague 'human activities', while the *NGO Alternative Treaty* and *Youth '92* identify specific activities and conditions such as the construction of large dams, unequal access to natural resources and the activities of multinational corporations.

Major points of comparison among the agendas

NGOs recognize the need for and make a commitment to political action. This is not found in *Agenda 21*. *Youth '92* and *Agenda 21* acknowledge that increasing pressure on land is leading to degradation, including desertification. *Agenda 21* points a rather non-specific finger at expanding human require-ments and economic activities while *Youth '92* specifically criticizes multinationals and developments such as large dams. The two agendas also stress the need for soil conservation. *Youth '92* suggests that this requires the phasing out of pesticides and fertilizers. *Youth '92* prefers small-scale projects to reduce land degradation.

Five years later

The biggest news in the area of desertification is that the Convention to Combat Desertification and Drought came into force on 26 December 1996. Chapter 12 of *Agenda 21* is generally credited with being the backbone of the Convention to Combat Desertification and Drought. As the Convention has only been in force for less than a year, it is hard to point to specific progress, although there are some positive signs. The International NGO Network on Desertification and Drought reports[47] that there is widespread development of national co-ordinating mechanisms. People from government institutions, NGOs, community-based organizations and at the grassroots level are begin-ning to talk with each other – some for the first time. Many countries have already established their National Coordinating Committees to oversee the development and implementation of the National Action Programmes.

At the regional level, countries are talking about shared resources and regional co-operation. Most regions now have had at least one regional con-ference involving governments and NGOs to discuss the implementation of the convention.

At the local level considerable work is being done to raise awareness of the convention and to prepare people for the National Action Programme process. One of the most notable successes of the convention has been the genuine acceptance by most governments of the need to develop a bottom-up approach. This change in attitude has brought NGOs much more into focus for govern-ments.

Energy

Caring for the Earth	chapter 10: Energy
Women's Action Agenda 21	Nuclear Power and Alternative Energy
Global Assembly of Women	Energy
Youth Action Guide	chapter 12: Energy
Changing Course	chapter 3: Energy and the Marketplace

Due to the lobbying efforts of a number of governments with a significant financial stake in the oil business, energy received scant attention in *Agenda 21*. The negative effects of unsustainable energy consumption, particularly the use of non-renewable energy sources in transportation and industrial development, were apparent at the time of UNCED. This fact was not lost on those who prepared the other agendas. Even the *UN Framework Convention on Climate Change*, which was signed during UNCED, emphasized the need to move away from dependence on fossil fuels to an environmentally friendly mix of carbon-free and renewable energy sources.

The agendas which look at energy agree that it is currently produced and consumed inefficiently and that the burning of fossil fuels causes air pollution. The *Women's Action Agenda 21* and *Global Assembly of Women* underline the risks of nuclear energy. The *Youth Action Guide* points out that many people cannot fulfil basic energy needs, and *Changing Course* identifies short-term planning by business and governments as one cause of energy problems. All agendas also recognize that *per capita* energy consumption is far higher in industrialized countries and that existing development models rely heavily on fossil fuels.

The fact that energy use also provides numerous benefits makes it a difficult issue to resolve. All agendas agree that the solution lies in increasing the efficiency of energy production and consumption and increasing the use of renewable sources.

Five years later

After receiving scant attention in *Agenda 21*, energy has emerged as one of the priority issues in the move towards global sustainability. The UNGASS review notes:

> energy is essential to economic and social development and improved quality of life . . . advances towards sustainable energy use are taking place and all parties can benefit from progress made in other countries . . . to advance this work at the intergovernmental level, the Commission on Sustainable Development will discuss energy issues at its ninth session.

Reviews in 1997 by organizations such as the Worldwatch Institute,[48] Energy 21[49] and the Global Energy Observatory[50] present evidence of progress in the sustainable energy sector but this is not directly linked to any of the agendas which appeared at the time of UNCED.

Land resources

Agenda 21   chapter 10: Integrated Approach to the Planning and Management of Land Resources/chapter 12: Combating Desertification and Drought

Youth '92   Protection of Natural Resources: Land, Soil, Desertification

Land resources are singled out only in *Agenda 21* and *Youth '92*. In *Youth '92* land is considered along with soil and desertification, while *Agenda 21* gives desertification a separate chapter.

Major points of comparison between the agendas

Both documents acknowledge that increasing pressure on land resources is leading to land degradation, including desertification. *Agenda 21* blames expanding human requirements and economic activities for land degradation. *Youth '92* is more specific, criticizing activities by multinationals and developments such as large dam projects. The two agendas also stress the need for soil conservation. *Youth '92* suggests that this will mean phasing out pesticides and fertilizers. *Youth '92* also supports small-scale rather than large-scale projects to reduce land degradation. This issue is not raised in chapters 10 or 12 of *Agenda 21*, and neither is *Youth '92*'s commitment to campaign for an immediate halt to waste dumping in developing countries.

Five years later

More specific and related issues such as agriculture and desertification are still prominent but land resources is not an issue that continues to be discussed in the global arena five years after UNCED.

Marine environment

Agenda 21	chapter 17: Protection of the Oceans, All Kinds of Seas, including Enclosed and Semi-enclosed Seas and Coastal Areas and the Protection, Rational Use and Development of their Living Resources
NGO Alternative Treaties	Fisheries Treaty, Pollution of the Marine Environment, Minimizing Physical Alteration of Marine Ecosystems, Protecting the Sea from Global Atmospheric Changes, Marine Biodiversity Treaty, Marine Protected Areas
ASCEND 21	chapter 8: Marine and Coastal Systems
Caring for the Earth	chapter 16: Oceans and Coastal Areas

Even before UNCED, the nature of the oceans forced the international community to look at problems in a global context, as evidenced by the *International Law of the Seas Agreement*.

Three agendas identify degradation of oceans and coastal environments as a pressing problem (*Agenda 21*, *ASCEND 21*, *Caring for the Earth*). *ASCEND 21* goes on to emphasize the importance of understanding the 'dynamic properties of the land–ocean interface'. The six *NGO Alternative Treaties* dealing with marine matters focus on the effects of a deteriorating ocean environment including the problems fishermen face from depleted fish stocks and toxic accumulations in the marine food chain.

Neither *Agenda 21* nor *ASCEND 21* gives specific causes for the oceans' problems, but *Caring for the Earth* and the *NGO Alternative Treaties* both point to human activities on land and sea which give rise to pollution and habitat destruction. The *NGO Alternative Treaties* lay the blame on mismanagement of coastal zones and ocean uses 'driven by an economic global model based on exploitation and generation of large profits'.

Major points of comparison among the agendas

Agenda 21's lengthy and comprehensive chapter 17 covers no fewer than six *NGO Alternative Treaties*. The problems and activities are identified in a very similar manner in both documents although the NGOs put much more emphasis on lobbying for change and action in problem areas. One major difference is the NGOs' emphasis on fishing as a livelihood. This is only mentioned in *Agenda 21*.

ASCEND 21 and *Agenda 21* name degradation of marine and coastal environments as the overall problem, although neither document identifies the reasons in a straightforward manner. Proposed activities are similar but only *Agenda 21* considers small island states, while *ASCEND 21* focuses on enhancing the scientific basis for action and explaining the present state of scientific knowledge on these issues.

Caring for the Earth and *Agenda 21* also propose similar activities such as controlling land-to-sea pollution, enforcing existing legislation and international conventions, recognizing the rights of small-scale users of fisheries and improving the monitoring of marine resources. *Caring for the Earth* urges an ecosystem approach to planning and advocates campaigning and lobbying on coastal and marine issues.

Five years later

The United Nations General Assembly Special Session on progress since the Earth Summit recognizes that there have been some positive developments in important areas of the marine environment. But there is still a great deal more that needs to be accomplished. They state that

> progress has been achieved since UNCED in the negotiation of agreements and voluntary instruments for improving the conservation and management of fishery resources and for the protection of the marine environment. Furthermore, progress has been made in the conservation and management of specific fishery stocks for securing the

sustainable utilization of these resources. Despite this, the decline of many fish stocks, high levels of discards, and rising marine pollution continue.

The International Oceans Institute reports that the conditions for being consistent with the guidelines in *Agenda 21* do not yet exist. The sustainable development of oceans requires

> [a] system of governance at the local, national, regional and global levels that is comprehensive, consistent, interdisciplinary, trans-sectoral, and participatory – bottom-up not top-down. The design of such a system should fully utilize existing institutions and abstain from creating new bureaucracies and additional financial burdens.[51]

Nuclear issues

Agenda 21	chapter 22: Safe and Environmentally Sound Management of Radioactive Waste
NGO Alternative Treaties	Treaty on the Nuclear Problem
Agenda Ya Wananchi	Appeal to Governments: End Nuclear Power/Weaponry Related Activities
Women's Action Agenda 21	Nuclear Power and Alternative Energy

All of the agendas that deal with nuclear issues focus on the dangers of radioactive waste. *Agenda 21* emphasizes the need for stringent protection measures but the other agendas (*NGO Alternative Treaty*, *Agenda Ya Wananchi*, the *Women's Action Agenda 21*) advocate stopping waste at the source by eliminating nuclear energy and nuclear weapons. The *Women's Action Agenda 21* points out the vulnerability of women and children to radiation-induced cancers.

Only the *NGO Alternative Treaty on the Nuclear Problem* offers a reason for the current use of nuclear power: the military nuclear industrial complex.

Major points of comparison among the agendas

There are important differences between *Agenda 21* and the *NGO Alternative Treaty*. *Agenda 21* focuses almost exclusively on waste issues, such as policies and programmes for its safe transport and storage, but does not address the issue of reducing the use of nuclear energy. The *NGO Alternative Treaty* stresses the potential dangers associated with nuclear energy and urges the use of alternative fuels. Both documents strongly discourage the export of radioactive waste.

Agenda Ya Wananchi takes a broader look at the nuclear issue, taking into account research, testing and use of nuclear technologies, and calling for an end to nuclear research and the use of all nuclear facilities. *Agenda 21* appears to accept the ongoing use of nuclear technology and focuses instead on controlling radioactive waste. The *Women's Action Agenda 21* also urges an end to the use of all nuclear technology.

Five years later

Many of the suggestions for the management of radioactive wastes made in *Agenda 21* were restated by UNGASS. They advised that 'further action is needed by the international community to address the need for enhancing awareness of the importance of safe management of radioactive wastes, and to ensure the prevention of incidents and accidents involving the uncontrolled release of such wastes'.

Science

Agenda 21	chapter 34: Technology Transfer/chapter 35: Science
ASCEND 21	chapter 13: Public Awareness, Science and the Environment
Women's Action Agenda 21	Science and Technology Transfer

The scientific community can play a leading role in ensuring that research programmes and related activities pursue the objectives agreed to at the Earth Summit. According to the International Council of Scientific Unions, this would require the integration of scientists from developing countries in sustainability research programmes as well as more cross-disciplinary work. The systematic nature of the problems we all face in the field of sustainable development makes it imperative that the search for solutions involve input from a range of disciplines, including the social, physical and life sciences.

Scientific research and innovation need not only a multidisciplinary perspective but also input from other groups including business, government and the non-governmental community. Scientific knowledge is produced through systematic observation, experiment and induction. The application of scientific knowledge can be crucial to understanding whether systems, be they social or ecological, are moving towards or away from sustainability. Scientific investigation can also uncover effective ways to dismantle barriers to the implementation of sustainability.

Three agendas consider science in the context of environment and development. Overall, *Agenda 21* and *ASCEND 21* stress scientists' role in providing information for decision-making (*Agenda 21*) and the need for science to help raise public awareness about environmental problems. The *Women's Action Agenda 21* says women are 'victimized by the misuse of scientific discoveries' and links the discussion of science with technology transfer.

Major points of comparison among the agendas

ASCEND 21 and *Agenda 21* address education and science from different perspectives. *Agenda 21* emphasizes the role scientists can play in providing information for decision-making concerning environment and development policy, while *ASCEND 21* indicates that scientists need to clarify their role in increasing awareness of environmental problems. Proposed activities in the two main chapters on education and science illustrate these divergent approaches. The role of science outlined in chapter 14 (Capacity Building) of *ASCEND 21* is closer to the more traditional discussion of the contribution the scientific community can make by sharing knowledge and increasing participation in decision-making.

Agenda 21 considers the benefits of technology and science, while the *Women's Action Agenda 21* focuses on how lack of access and misuse of technology and scientific discoveries have a negative impact on women. The *Women's Action Agenda 21* sees the underlying problem as the detachment of ethical values from research.

Five years later

This topic was not addressed in a major way in the UNGASS review. However, in early 1997 the International Council of Scientific Unions conducted its own review of the implementation of the recommendations from *ASCEND 21*, many of which are similar to those presented in *Agenda 21*. They concluded that there had been progress in four main areas, including:

- strengthened cohesion and co-operation between scientific groups in different countries and across disciplines;
- enhanced communication and co-operation with decision-makers and end-users of research;
- involvement of economics and the social sciences in global research programmes; and
- enhanced data accessibility.

Technology

Agenda 21	chapter 34: Transfer of Environmentally Sound Technology, Co-operation and Capacity Building
NGO Alternative Treaties	Treaty on a Technology Bank Solidarity System for Technological Exchange
Agenda Ya Wananchi	Technology Transfer
ASCEND 21	chapter 15: Policies for Technology
Women's Action Agenda 21	Science and Technology Transfer

Global Assembly of Women	Environmentally-friendly Systems, Products and Technologies
Youth Action Guide	chapter 10: Appropriate Technology and Technology Transfer
Changing Course	chapter 8: Technology Co-operation

The most pressing issue in this area is access to technology, including environmentally sound technology (*Agenda 21*), needed technology (*Agenda Ya Wananchi*), appropriate and sustainable technology (the *Women's Action Agenda 21*) and technologies which will allow nations to make better use of their resources (the *Youth Action Guide*). There is also agreement on the importance of developing technologies based on traditional knowledge (*Agenda Ya Wananchi*) and indigenous methods (*Global Assembly of Women*) and the need to support economic development and growth with clean and efficient technology (*ASCEND 21, Changing Course*).

A number of intellectual and practical reasons are given for current barriers to environmental technology. They include failure to understand the nature of change (*ASCEND 21*), separation of ethical values from scientific investigation and use (the *Women's Action Agenda 21*) and a concept development based on natural resources (*NGO Alternative Treaty*).

Major points of comparison among the agendas

There is agreement on the need for increased access to technology, but the *NGO Alternative Treaty* insists that the technology be pragmatic, accessible and culturally and socially compatible. *Agenda 21* focuses on facilitating the transfer of technology but is not as specific on parameters. Both documents recommend the establishment of an international technology bank.

There is a high degree of conformity between *Agenda 21* and *Agenda Ya Wananchi* in this area. Both recognize the need for greater access to environmentally sound technologies and the importance of indigenous technologies. *ASCEND 21* emphasizes the improvement of science and technology policy, and recognition of the links between environmental and economic imperatives. The documents present similar approaches to capacity building and emphasize the importance of creating conditions which encourage local innovation. The technology chapter in *ASCEND 21* is presented in a particularly expansive essay style providing historical and philosophical background to the technology transfer debate.

The issue of technology is addressed differently in *Agenda 21* and the *Global Assembly of Women*. *Agenda 21* looks at access to and transfer of environmentally sound technology, while the *Global Assembly of Women* focuses on the re-introduction of indigenous technologies for waste management and natural resource protection. Women are urged to use their power as consumers to achieve desired goals.

The *Youth Action Guide* raises the issue of the environmental technology requirements of small business. It also emphasizes activities involving youth, such as internship programmes and including indigenous youth in the implementation of technology.

Agenda 21 and *Changing Course* agree about the need for wider access to environmentally sound technologies but *Changing Course* links this more strongly to minimum or non-polluting and equitable economic growth. Both agendas see the primary method of improving access to technology as 'moving technology from where it exists to where it is needed'. Both also underline the need to respect patents and intellectual property rights and to recognize the requirements of and contributions from local communities. *Agenda 21* and *Changing Course* also agree on the 'special role' of multinational companies in facilitating technology transfer.

Five years later

The UNGASS review restated many of the objectives for technology transfer outlined in *Agenda 21*. There was no clear indication that much progress had been made, evidenced by statements such as 'there is an urgent need for developing countries to acquire greater access to environmentally sound technologies if they are to meet the obligations agreed at UNCED'.

The World Business Council on Sustainable Development was able to identify some progress on the recommendations contained in *Changing Course*. The examples presented in *Signals of Change* emphasized increasing access to technology through technology co-operation. 'Simply giving new technologies to those who need it . . . has been shown to be ineffective'. Examples of joint ventures and technology co-operation since 1992 include cases such as these:

> about 100 managers from the Ministry of Electric Power in China participating in an exchange program with the Tokyo Electric Power Company, concentrating on proper and effective operation and management, including environmental consciousness raising. In South America, Northern Telecom of Canada has worked with the US and Mexican Governments to tackle ozone depletion by devising new ways to eliminate the use of chlorofluorocarbons in Mexican industry.

The WBCSD also cites South–South technology co-operation, including 'BCSD Colombia helping small companies involved in highly polluting manufacturing, such as the leather business, to cut pollution through ways that save money'.

Waste management

Agenda 21	chapter 21: Environmentally Sound Management of Solid Wastes and Sewage-related Issues
NGO Alternative Treaties	Treaty on Waste
ASCEND 21	chapter 3: Industry and Waste
Global Assembly of Women	Waste
Youth Action Guide	chapter 13: Waste Management

This topic covers many different kinds of wastes, from household garbage, much of which may be suitable for municipal recycling programmes, to toxic by-products of industrial processes. Wastes such as polychlorinated biphenols (PCBs), which do not break down easily, if at all, and can therefore become concentrated in the food chain, are known as persistent organic pollutants (POPs). In general, the sustainable management of all wastes is linked to changes in existing production and consumption methodologies and patterns.

All of the agendas dealing with waste emphasize the connection between the production of waste and environmental degradation. The *Global Assembly of Women* also mentions the build-up of waste resulting from a failure to consider waste as a potential resource. The generation of large quantities of waste results from unsustainable patterns of consumption and production (*Agenda 21*) and an economic development model in which 'society as a whole, and the poor in particular, suffer from the economic costs of soil, water and food contamination as well as air pollution' (*NGO Alternative Treaty*). Other suggested causes include an inability to maximize process efficiency and use waste as a resource, consumer acceptance of waste-generating products and over-packaging, lack of penalties for waste generation (*Youth Action Guide*) and continued reliance on virgin raw materials and fossil fuels (*ASCEND 21*).

Major points of comparison among the agendas

Agenda 21 and the *NGO Alternative Treaty on Waste* are similar in a number of respects including their recognition of the links between many waste-related issues – for example, *Agenda 21* suggests consulting the chapters on freshwater, human settlement, protection and promotion of human health and changing consumption – and encouraging sound waste management such as recycling and re-use. The NGO document also urges political pressure to achieve the stated goals.

ASCEND 21 focuses on waste from industry, using a broad definition of industry that includes the 'sum total of materials/energy transformational activities . . . including extractive industries and final consumption wastes'. Most of the recommendations in *ASCEND 21* are the same as those of *Agenda 21*, although the science agenda places greater emphasis on research into areas such as raw materials substitution. While *Agenda 21* and the *Global Assembly of Women* both advocate recycling, the *Global Assembly of Women* emphasizes the need for responsible consumer behaviour whereas *Agenda 21* sees more value in encouraging management practices such as waste minimization, cleaner production technologies and recycling. The *Youth Action Guide* considers these same issues but proposes more activities involving industry, communities and individuals. The *Youth Action Guide* also suggests 'penalizing industry and households' according to the quantity and toxicity of the waste they produce. This inducement to change is not found in *Agenda 21*.

Five years later

Although much remains to be done to implement the recommendations in *Agenda 21* relating to waste, the UNGASS review felt that 'substantial progress on the sound management of chemicals has been made since UNCED'. They cite the establishment of the Intergovernmental Forum on Chemical Safety (IFCS) and the Inter-Organizational Programme for the Sound Management of Chemicals (IOMC)'.

Water

Agenda 21	chapter 18: Protection of the Quality and Supply of Freshwater Resources
NGO Alternative Treaties	Freshwater Treaty
ASCEND 21	chapter 10: Freshwater Resources
Caring for the Earth	chapter 15: Freshwaters
Global Assembly of Women	Water
Youth '92	Protection of Natural Resources: Water Resources
Voice of the Eagle	Water
Changing Course	chapter 10: Leadership for Sustainable Development in Developing Countries

The three issues which dominate the discussion on water (also called freshwater in some agendas) are water pollution, scarcity of water and lack of access to freshwater.

Major points of comparison among the agendas

Agenda 21 emphasizes specific activities for alleviating freshwater scarcity and pollution, while *ASCEND 21* puts greater emphasis on scientific analysis and research.

Caring for the Earth and *Agenda 21* take similar approaches, identifying the increasing scarcity and pollution of freshwater as major problems. The two documents also agree that an increase in activities which are incompatible with protecting and sustaining freshwater resources lie at the heart of the problem. Many of the proposed activities are the same. Both agendas recognize the need for increased public participation in decision-making on freshwater, with *Caring for the Earth* putting a greater emphasis on local community management. *Agenda 21* sees a need to find mechanisms for North–South co-operation on water problems.

The *Global Assembly of Women* highlights the need for universal access to clean water, while *Agenda 21* concentrates on the causes of water pollution. The accompanying suggestions for actions in *Agenda 21*, therefore, focus on preventing or eliminating water pollution, while the *Global Assembly of Women* focuses on water availability and distribution.

Water resource contamination and depletion are identified as important problems by both *Agenda 21* and *Youth '92*. The two agendas also agree that an increase in activities incompatible with high water quality is the underlying cause. *Youth '92* goes further in listing the incompatible activities (such as mining, agro-chemical use, deforestation, military nuclear testing). The two documents propose more community involvement in the management of water resources, and *Agenda 21* stresses the importance of ensuring universal access to good water.

Voice of the Eagle states that no one should be allowed to own water. *Agenda 21* proposes many technical activities such as twinning North–South research centres and reducing the prevalence of water-borne disease. These technical approaches are not found in *Voice of the Eagle*. Instead, water is referred to as 'the life blood of Mother Earth', 'a life-giving force' and prophecies about future scarcity of freshwater and associated fighting and loss of life are cited.

Changing Course focuses on the lack of access to freshwater and highlights the role that international corporations can play in increasing the availability of water through technology co-operation. *Changing Course* also considers the problem from the perspective of those who are able to pay for water and those who are not. This market-orientated angle of analysis is not dealt with in *Agenda 21*.

Five years later

Following UNCED, the CSD set up the Global Water Assessment, which issued a major report in 1997. Findings did not yet indicate widespread improvement in this area and recommendations were made for greater national and international co-ordination.

6

AGENDA 21 AND OTHER SUSTAINABLE DEVELOPMENT AGENDAS

Agenda 21 covers more topics than any other agenda in this study. It is the only one that emphasizes the role of United Nations organizations in achieving a more sustainable way of living. It also places greater emphasis on actions that do not challenge national sovereignty. It is more conservative than many of the agendas in the degree of change it advocates but it also represents more people than any other agenda.

This chapter compares *Agenda 21* with each of the agendas used in this study, taking into account differences and similarities in objectives, principles, priorities and actions.

Agenda 21 and the *NGO Alternative Treaties*

The overall objectives and principles of *Agenda 21* and the *NGO Alternative Treaties* are articulated most clearly in the declarations signed by the two groups. The Rio Declaration on Environment and Development represents the basic principles underlying *Agenda 21* and was agreed to by all signatories to *Agenda 21*. The NGOs put forward three declarations (the Earth Charter, People's Earth Declaration and the Rio Declaration on Environment and Development) that outline the spirit behind the *NGO Alternative Treaties* ratified at Rio as well as presenting an ethical framework for future NGO activities.

Similarities

Parties to *Agenda 21* and the *NGO Alternative Treaties* agree on many objectives for a more environmentally sustainable world. These include:

- eradication of poverty;
- assumption of greater responsibility by industrialized countries for current environmental problems;
- elimination of over-consumption and unsustainable production of goods;
- increased access to information;

- enhanced democratic participation in decision-making;
- development based on the 'precautionary principle';
- acknowledgement of the importance of indigenous peoples and their knowledge and traditional practices for achieving sustainable development;
- full participation of women to achieve sustainable development;
- recognition of the interrelated nature of environment, development and peace; and
- international co-operation of nations and people to achieve the stated objectives.

Differences

Sometimes the Rio Declaration on Environment and Development and the various NGO declarations place different emphasis on similar topics; sometimes they make completely distinct statements. Many of these distinctions reflect the nature of UN activities such as ensuring the sovereign rights of nations, working towards international agreements and standards, notifying other states when natural disasters occur, notification of transboundary effects, respecting international law and peacefully resolving environmental disputes in accordance with the Charter of the UN. All are principles contained in the Rio Declaration on Environment and Development.

In general, these principles are not given primary importance by the NGO declarations, which concentrate on broader ethical, social and ecological principles. They recognize the need for change in many areas: acknowledging the limits to natural capital, recognizing the diversity of life on the planet, incorporating gender balance in planning and action, the requirement for a new economic system that serves the needs of the many in an equitable manner, changing to alternative energy sources, and formulating a transparent and clearly articulated ethical basis for development.

Clarifying and acknowledging values is particularly prominent throughout the *NGO Alternative Treaties* with an entire treaty (Ethical Commitments) devoted to the subject. This emphasis on ethics is missing from *Agenda 21* and is one of the major distinctions between the two sets of documents. *Agenda 21* does, however, indicate the need to question current values (for example, chapter 4.11: 'consideration should also be given to the present concepts of economic growth and the need for new concepts of wealth and prosperity which allow higher standards of living and are less dependent on the Earth's finite resources').

The most obvious difference between the two sets of documents lies in how they propose to proceed in attacking the identified problems. The NGOs make a clear commitment to work towards removing the injustices in the current world socio-economic system (for instance, Treaty on Alternative Economic Models). In *Agenda 21*, on the other hand, there appears to be a tacit acceptance of the need to work, primarily although not exclusively, within the existing system. Many chapters cite existing international agreements which need to be enforced or implemented in order to achieve the objectives defined in that chapter (for example, chapter 9, Protection of the Atmosphere: 1985 Vienna Convention for the Protection of the Ozone Layer; 1987 Montreal Protocol on Substances that Deplete the Ozone Layer, as amended; 1992 United Nations Convention on Climate Change). This fundamental difference in perspective is most apparent when considering how the two sets of documents explain the causes of current environment and development problems.

Reason for the problem

On many issues, *Agenda 21* and the *NGO Alternative Treaties* define the general problems in a similar manner (for example, urbanization – the need to address deterioration of human settlement conditions; decision-making – the need to strengthen democratic participation; atmosphere – the need for a better understanding of the impacts of ozone depletion and an increase in atmospheric greenhouse gases). In these cases the primary difference lies in identifying the underlying cause of the problem. In general, *Agenda 21* either does not discuss causes or presents them in a straightforward way (for instance, 12.2, desertification is the result of climatic variations and human activities). The *NGO Alternative Treaties* tend to 'lay the blame', citing, for example, interlinking factors such as current development and consumption patterns, powerful and unaccountable transnational corporations, equity issues such as unequal access to natural resources, social injustice and the existing dominant model of economic development.

Proposed actions

Another broad distinction between the *NGO Alternative Treaties* and *Agenda 21* is the level at which action is suggested. Not surprisingly, given the parties involved in the negotiation, *Agenda 21* emphasizes action at the national or governmental level. The *NGO Alternative Treaties* stress personal commitment for change. Both documents agree on the importance of input and participation at the local and community level.

Many of the *NGO Alternative Treaties* summarize commitments made by the signatories (for instance, *Alternative Treaty on Climate Change* – act in solidarity with other NGOs; inform and support NGOs working on this issue). The treaties emphasize the need for organizing and lobbying for political change. This approach to action is missing from *Agenda 21*.

Agenda 21 is a much longer document and includes more specific suggestions for sustainable development activities (for example, Urbanization – 7.69, 'develop policies and practices to reach the informal sector and self-help housing builders by adopting measures to increase the affordability of building materials on the part of the urban and rural poor, through, *inter alia*, credit schemes and bulk procurement of building materials for sale to small-scale builders and communities'). However, it is also rife with vague suggestions such as 'increase collaboration', 'open up the decision-making process' and 'strengthen the sustainable development component of all planning programmes'.

Agenda 21 and *Agenda Ya Wananchi*

The principles and objectives which are central to *Agenda Ya Wananchi* are found in the first section of the document, which includes a preamble, a list of principles and three small essays on, respectively, the current world order, the global crisis and the people's response.

Similarities

There are few direct similarities between the two documents, partly because they use such different language but also because economic development is only mentioned in *Agenda Ya Wananchi* but plays a major role in the objectives and actions of *Agenda 21*. On fundamental principles, however, the two agendas agree on the following points:

- the needs of future generations must be considered in current planning;
- eradication of poverty is an extremely important and urgent responsibility of humankind;
- a global partnership is necessary to achieve environmental change;
- the industrialized world is responsible for many current environmental problems;
- unsustainable patterns of consumption are responsible for many social and environmental problems;
- citizens need to take a greater role in decision-making;
- the precautionary principle should be used during decision-making; and
- women need to play a greater role in environmental management.

Differences

The different goals of the two agendas are reflected in the language used to describe existing social and environmental issues, in the issues given priority, in recommended actions and in the stated principles and objectives.

Agenda Ya Wananchi emphasizes the transition to 'a more socially just and environmentally secure world'. Although no principal goal is specified in the Rio Declaration or *Agenda 21*, a recurring theme is 'integration of environment and development concerns' to lead to 'the fulfilment of basic needs, improved standards of living for all, better protected and managed ecosystems and a safer and more prosperous future' (chapter 1, Preamble).

75

This emphasis on development and prosperity is not found in *Agenda Ya Wananchi*, which gives prominence to protecting cultural diversity, self-determination and restructuring society. In *Agenda 21* these topics are mentioned in passing, if at all. *Agenda Ya Wananchi* also repeatedly criticizes developed countries for wasteful and destructive practices that are the cause of most of the Earth's ecological problems, in the South and the North. Although the Rio Declaration recognizes the special needs of developing countries, it does not blame industrialized countries with the same vehemence.

Agenda Ya Wananchi suggests lifting the debt of poor countries. Although it is mentioned in the body of *Agenda 21*, debt is not found among the twenty-seven principles of the Rio Declaration and the idea of removing the debt of developing countries completely is never raised.

The two documents are very different with respect to priorities and actions. *Agenda Ya Wananchi* emphasizes the societal aspects of environment. Although social issues are considered in *Agenda 21*, they are far outweighed by considerations of physical/biological science and economics. Increasing prosperity and economic development are seen as unimportant, even undesirable, in *Agenda Ya Wananchi*. They are among the top priorities in *Agenda 21*, although they are to be pursued in tandem with sound environmental management.

Most of the actions proposed by *Agenda Ya Wananchi* are missing from *Agenda 21*. Numerous calls for campaigns, protests and commitments are the nature of many NGO documents and it is understandable that these are not found in *Agenda 21*, a document agreed to by representatives of national governments. *Agenda Ya Wananchi* urges a number of actions not found in *Agenda 21*, including preventing the patenting of life forms and genetic material, restricting the advertising of products which harm the environment, stopping all nuclear-related activities, allowing indigenous and tribal peoples the right to self-determination and ownership of pre-colonial lands and supporting alternative or fair trade over free trade.

Agenda 21 and *ASCEND 21*

The major principles and objectives underlying *Agenda 21* and *ASCEND 21* are very different. The Rio Declaration outlines broad objectives, including 'the goal of establishing new and equitable global partnership' and pursuing development 'to equitably meet development and environmental needs of present and future generations'. While the two documents raise many of the same issues and in many cases treat them similarly, *ASCEND 21* was undertaken to stimulate discussion in the scientific community (hence the emphasis on lengthy background material) while *Agenda 21* was directed at policy- and decision-makers at the national, regional and local levels.

Although *ASCEND 21* often goes further than *Agenda 21* in identifying broader philosophical grounds for a given situation (such as failure to understand the problem of change), there is much conformity with respect to defining problems and identifying the causes. In some instances, *ASCEND 21* puts greater emphasis on prevailing social conditions as an underlying cause (for example, over-consumption by wealthy nations – chapter 11; production and consumption associated with a growing population – chapter 7).

A major distinction between the two agendas is the quantity and nature of the specific activities proposed. *ASCEND 21* pays greater attention to explaining the current situation and suggesting activities where scientific understanding requires clarification. *Agenda 21* is much more prescription-orientated. *ASCEND 21* also contains the recurring theme that scientists 'have the responsibility to explain to the citizen and to policy-makers the importance of sustainable development to the well-being of the individual and the future of the society', although in chapter 13 (Public Awareness, Science and the Environment) scientists are cautioned to recognize the limitations 'of their own intellectual techniques and disciplines'.

Agenda 21 and *Caring for the Earth*

The principles and objectives behind *Caring for the Earth* are spelled out in the first chapter of the strategy for sustainable living, called 'Building a Sustainable Society'.

Similarities

The two documents share a number of the same major principles. These include the following:
- human beings are at the centre of concerns for sustainable development;
- there is a need for awareness of the effects of present actions on future generations;
- there is a need to reduce disparities in standards of living;
- economically poorer countries may require financial help for environmental protection and to develop in a sustainable manner. This is the responsibility of developed countries;
- there is a need for global partnership to achieve global sustainability;
- it is important to understand and keep production and consumption within the Earth's carrying capacity; and
- there is a need for increased participation in environment and development decision-making and an accompanying access to and dissemination of information.

Differences

The different goals of these documents reflect, naturally, the characteristics of those responsible for their development. The Rio Declaration was made by nation states, so there is greater emphasis on national government objectives and on various aspects of international relations, such as 'establishing a new and equitable global partnership through the creation of new levels of co-operation among states, key sectors of societies and people' and 'working towards international agreements which respect the interests of all and protect the integrity of the global environmental and developmental system'. *Caring for the Earth* was prepared by three international environmental organizations and the primary objectives involve improving the quality of human life while conserving 'the vitality and diversity of the Earth'.

These distinctions are also apparent in the stated principles of the two pieces of work. The Rio Declaration stresses matters of international concern such as notifying other nations of activities with trans-boundary effects and discouraging or preventing activities and substances that cause environmental degradation to other states. *Caring for the Earth* highlights the importance of community activities and changes in personal practices and attitudes. Like the *NGO Alternative Treaties*, *Caring for the Earth* places greater emphasis on ethical responsibilities than *Agenda 21* (for example, it states that it is essential to build public consensus around an ethic for living sustainably).

The Rio Declaration says that economic initiatives such as internalizing environmental costs and the 'polluter pays principle' are vital, while *Caring for the Earth* encourages national policies that relate economics to environmental carrying capacity. Respect for the Earth's carrying capacity is a more prevalent theme throughout *Caring for the Earth*.

The two documents identify many of the same important issues and propose many similar types of actions. However, whereas the actions suggested in *Agenda 21* range from the very general to the very specific, *Caring for the Earth* contains a higher proportion of specific activities and guidelines (such as proposed guidelines for sustainable industrial processes – Box 18). *Caring for the Earth* suggests that lobbying and political campaigns are necessary to bring about needed policy and lifestyle changes (for example, chapter 4 – Conserving the Earth's Vitality and Diversity; chapter 16 – Oceans and Coastal Areas). This approach is not found in *Agenda 21*. The diplomatic tone of much of *Agenda 21* means that a number of the controversial issues raised in *Caring for the Earth* are not addressed directly. These include intellectual property rights, family planning, government regulation of industrial activities and the failure of local and national governments to fulfil their obligations and responsibilities.

Caring for the Earth places a high priority on locally implemented solutions (such as local production of food to meet local needs), and gives greater consideration to integrating the numerous systems that contribute to environmental problems and solutions than is apparent in *Agenda 21*. While *Agenda 21* emphasizes improving understanding of various problems (like atmospheric processes), *Caring for the Earth* identifies the sources of those problems (for instance, global pollution, ecosystem destruction).

Agenda 21 and the Women's Action Agenda 21

The principles and objectives underlying the *Women's Action Agenda 21* are not specified in any one section although the basic context is set in the preamble, which touches on most of the major principles found throughout the document. The report of a tribunal made up of five supreme court justices from Guyana, Australia, India, Kenya and Sweden lists the three principles – global equity, resource ethics and empowerment of women – that must form the basis for the needed changes in the social and physical environment.

Similarities

The two agendas have little in common with respect to their stated principles, partly because their goals are different. The *Women's Action Agenda 21* is designed to highlight women's issues in the realm of environment and development. But most women's issues are also the issues facing all humankind, which is what *Agenda 21* attempts to address. Shared principles and objectives include:

- eradication of poverty;
- decreasing disparities in quality of life between rich and poor;
- ensuring full participation of women in environment and development;
- eliminating unsustainable patterns of production and consumption;
- ensuring greater participation of citizens in decision-making;
- respecting indigenous people and their lands.

Differences

The *Women's Action Agenda 21* emphasizes the role of women and the social aspects of the environment. *Agenda 21* devotes more space to the physical/biological environment, although it recognizes the links between various facets of the environments.

The *Women's Action Agenda 21* speaks clearly on the importance of moral and spiritual values, an emphasis missing from *Agenda 21*. It also criticizes the concepts of a 'free market' and 'economic growth', both of which are important objectives in *Agenda 21*. The *Women's Action Agenda 21* calls for self-determination for all peoples (including indigenous peoples) and points out the wastefulness and uselessness of violence and militarism in solving problems. These points are not found in *Agenda 21*.

Many of the priorities and actions found in *Agenda 21* are also present in the *Women's Action Agenda 21*, reflecting the success of the lobby based on the *Women's Action Agenda* in the UNCED negotiations. References to the special situation or needs of women resulting from inequitable policies and programmes are found in almost every chapter of *Agenda 21*.

Ethics, militarism and democratic rights are priority issues in the *Women's Action Agenda 21* that do not rank chapter or major issue status in *Agenda 21*. The *Women's Action Agenda 21* recognizes a strong link between biotechnology and biodiversity (for instance, the patenting of life forms in the South by companies from the North, threatening the natural biological heritage of the South), while *Agenda 21* covers them in separate chapters. The *Women's Action Agenda 21* places greater emphasis on the need for personal lifestyle changes (like using public transport instead of cars). Family planning is discussed in a straightforward manner in the *Women's Action Agenda 21* but only hinted at in *Agenda 21* (for example, 'reproductive health programmes and services should, as appropriate, be developed and enhanced . . . and enable women and men to fulfil their personal aspirations in terms of family size').

Two activities proposed by the *Women's Action Agenda 21* and not found at all in *Agenda 21* are the ending of the use of all nuclear technology and the cancellation of foreign debt in developing countries.

Agenda 21 and the *Global Assembly of Women and the Environment*

The primary goal of the *Global Assembly of Women* was 'to demonstrate women's capacity in environmental management, the elements of leadership necessary for success and the policies which can advance or retard such efforts'. The primary goal of the United Nations Conference on Environment and Development was to 'achieve sustainable development through the integration of environment and development goals' with *Agenda 21* expanding on this objective. The *Global Assembly of Women* focused on good environmental management rather than development. The principles behind *Agenda 21* are clearly laid out in the Rio Declaration, but there is no section in the *Global Assembly of Women* which explains the agenda's guiding principles.

With the exception of energy, themes covered in the *Global Assembly of Women* are also given chapter-level status in *Agenda 21*. Within the chapters and major recommendations similar actions are proposed. The *Global Assembly of Women* stresses the role of women as consumers and suggests more activities stemming from that role. It also considers technology in a broader sense to include environmentally friendly systems and products and sees greater significance in indigenous technologies and methodologies. Understandably, the *Global Assembly of Women* focuses on issues affecting women. The need for access to clean water is given greater attention than in *Agenda 21*, which concentrates on preventing or eliminating water contamination.

Agenda 21 and *Youth '92*

The objectives and principles of the World Youth Forum are outlined in the executive summary and introduction to *Youth '92*.

Similarities

The World Youth Forum from which the *Youth '92* document emerged centred on networking and exchange among young people active in environment and development issues. It also attempted to prepare young people for UNCED and the Global Forum including follow-up to these two events. However, another primary objective was to 'work for better understanding between the two parts of the world' – that is, between nations divided on economic and geographical grounds into North and South. This coincides with the Rio Declaration principle that nations need to 'co-operate in the spirit of global partnership to conserve, protect and restore the environment'. Other shared principles and objectives include:

- eradication of poverty;
- elimination of over-consumption;
- the necessity for greater participation of citizens to move towards a better world;
- involvement of youth in forming a global partnership for sustainable development;
- peaceful resolution by states of environmental disputes;
- special priority for the special needs of developing countries.

Differences

The different objectives and principles of the two documents reflect different views about who is to blame for the most serious environmental and development problems. The Rio Declaration does acknowledge that developed countries have a special responsibility in 'pursuit of sustainable development in view of the pressures their societies place on the global environment and of the technologies and financial resources they command'. *Youth '92*, however, places the blame for many specific problems such as poverty, debt and over-consumption squarely on the shoulders of the North.

Agenda 21 attempts to address as many environment and development issues as possible, while *Youth '92* deliberately confines itself to areas that will promote understanding between North and South. However, many issues which are given separate chapters in *Agenda 21* are components of one of the five major themes of *Youth '92*. Biodiversity and biotechnology, for example, are closely linked in *Youth '92* but are separate subjects in *Agenda 21*, reflecting a different perspective on the interrelated nature of the problems.

The agendas also differ on the reasons for certain environment and development problems. *Youth '92* refers repeatedly to the unsustainable practices of Northern companies and societies as well as multinational corporations, while *Agenda 21* is much less specific or certain. *Youth '92* accepts that climate change has already begun, while *Agenda 21* calls for greater understanding of what causes change in atmospheric conditions.

Youth '92 proposes a number of actions which are not found in *Agenda 21*, including regulating the activities of transnational corporations, prohibiting the patenting of genetically engineered organisms, cancelling the foreign debt of developing countries, halting the dumping of all foreign waste in countries of the South and strict regulation of biotechnology research, development and implementation.

Agenda 21 and the *Youth Action Guide on Sustainable Development*

The fundamental objectives of the *Youth Action Guide* are laid out in the introduction and in chapter 1. *Agenda 21* focuses on moving towards improved integration of environment and development for the 'fulfilment of basic needs, improved standards of living for all, better protected and managed ecosystems and a safer and more prosperous future' (chapter 1, Preamble). The *Youth Action Guide* has similar goals but concentrates on fulfilling youth's role in sustainable development. This concurs with Principle 21 of the Rio Declaration, which states: 'The creativity, ideals and courage of the youth of the world should be mobilised to forge a global partnership in order to achieve sustainable development and ensure a better future for all.'

Differences

Although the goal is sustainable development, the two documents differ on several fundamental objectives. The *Youth Action Guide*'s objectives are not necessarily at odds with *Agenda 21* but they are stated more clearly. They include the following:

- there is an urgent need to change the current world situation;
- youth need to lobby for legislation to protect the future and to act against those who are currently exploiting environmental resources;
- sustainable development must become an accepted element in the management of resources;
- youth must gain acceptance from other sectors of society to be part of forming a new sustainable way of life;
- fundamental changes are necessary in value systems and the day-to-day lives of individuals.

Throughout the *Youth Action Guide* there is a call to 'personalize' suggested actions by changing lifestyles and questioning existing conditions. This focus on personal commitment is not found in *Agenda 21*.

Agenda 21 and the *Youth Action Guide* have similar perspectives on many issues, including technology, deforestation, trade and business and industry. The *Youth Action Guide* stresses pricing policies and economic incentives as instruments of change (for example, high taxes on environmentally unfriendly products, economic incentives to protect forests) more strongly than *Agenda 21*. The *Youth Action Guide* also considers implications and possibilities for small businesses more fully than *Agenda 21* and is more critical of 'irresponsible actions by multinationals'. The *Youth Action Guide* is more direct in advocating family planning and offers more specific suggestions for preventing the spread of AIDS.

Many of the physical environment topics given priority in *Agenda 21* (such as freshwater, marine environment, biodiversity) are not addressed in the *Youth Action Guide*. However, the editors point out in the introduction that 'sustainable development covers all facets of human activity and, obviously, we have not been able to cover everything in this guide'. In contrast, *Agenda 21* is much more wide-reaching.

Agenda 21 and *Voice of the Eagle*

Voice of the Eagle wants to warn the inhabitants of the world that 'the sacredness of Mother Earth is not being respected'. Although the Rio Declaration and *Agenda 21* have no stated overall goal, a recurring theme is 'integration of environment and development concerns' to lead to 'the fulfilment of basic needs, improved standards of living for all, better protected and managed ecosystems and a safer and more prosperous future' (chapter 1, Preamble). These themes are not in direct opposition to *Voice of the Eagle* but neither are they entirely complementary. Economic conditions are not a priority in *Voice of the Eagle*. Prosperity and standards of living are not mentioned. Rather, the focus is on 'listening to the spiritual voice of the Eagle' and recognizing that 'Mother Earth does not belong to us – we belong to Mother Earth'.

The language of the two documents is also different. In *Agenda 21* terms such as 'awareness' have a technical meaning, such as awareness of relevant information. In *Voice of the Eagle* awareness generally refers to spiritual awareness or awareness of one's own part of a greater whole.

There is little common ground between the principles of *Agenda 21* as stated in the Rio Declaration and the principles found throughout *Voice of the Eagle*. The concept of development is central to the objectives and principles of *Agenda 21*. In *Voice of the Eagle* love is emphasized throughout the stated principles and the whole document. The word 'love' is not found in the Rio Declaration or in *Agenda 21*. The first three principles of each document illustrate this difference in emphasis.

Rio Declaration on Environment and Development	Voice of the Eagle
• Human beings are at the centre of sustainable development • States have a right to exploit their sustainable development • The rights of development must be fulfilled to meet development and environment needs of future and present generations equitably	• All life exists as an expression of the Creator's love • The greatest teaching and medicine in the world is love • To the indigenous peoples, Eagle symbolizes the power of the Creator's love

Improving humankind's relationship with the natural environment is a priority in both documents but the actions proposed for doing this are very different. In fact, *Voice of the Eagle* does not suggest actions, as such, but instead encourages a fundamental change in personal attitude to achieve greater harmony within the environment. In *Voice of the Eagle* proposals for change are presented in a non-demanding way, as if any just and sensible person, upon being made aware of the current state of social and environmental disruption, would naturally alter his or her behaviour. *Agenda 21* concentrates on policy-making and programme implementation.

Voice of the Eagle suggests raising children to be sensitive to and have respect for their relationship to other living things as part of nature. Child-rearing is not mentioned in *Agenda 21*. *Voice of the Eagle* also speaks out against pharmaceutical companies making profits from the knowledge of indigenous medicine people, another issue not considered in *Agenda 21*.

Agenda 21 and *Changing Course*

The fundamental principles underpinning *Changing Course* are presented at the beginning of the book in the Declaration of the Business Council for Sustainable Development.

Similarities

The documents are the products of agreements within two different groups: namely, government and business leaders. However, they share a number of the same underlying principles, including the following:

• the needs of the present must be met without compromising the welfare of future generations;
• environmental protection must be integrated into the development process;
• a spirit of co-operation is needed to achieve the goals of sustainable development;

- poverty must be alleviated;
- awareness must be increased and changes encouraged towards more sustainable patterns of consumption;
- participation in decision-making relating to the environment must be broadened;
- open trade policies and practices should be supported;
- a transfer of technology should occur from those who have it to those who need it;
- actions should be based on the precautionary principle; and
- environmental costs should be internalized.

Differences

The major differences in the principles articulated in the two documents stem from the fact that *Agenda 21* is concerned with the role of governments in achieving sustainable development while *Changing Course* focuses on business. *Changing Course* accepts the premise that 'economic growth is essential' to alleviate problems such as poverty and unsustainable population growth. The benefits of economic growth, *per se*, are not advanced as strongly in *Agenda 21*. Where *Changing Course* highlights the need for more efficient use and recovery of resources, the Rio Declaration stresses 'the sovereign right' of states to 'exploit their own resources pursuant to their own environmental and development policies'.

Agenda 21 and *Changing Course* agree on most of the priorities and actions that are addressed in both documents. *Changing Course* sometimes focuses more strongly on the human dimensions of issues such as population, where fulfilling basic human needs is highlighted, and freshwater, where access to uncontaminated water is given prominence. *Agenda 21* concentrates on the planet's resources and the increasing scarcity of freshwater. Poverty also is approached differently, with *Agenda 21* looking at income distribution and poor development of human resources while *Changing Course* sees poverty as a consequence of rapid urbanization.

The role of markets in alleviating environmental problems is more prominent throughout *Changing Course*. Understandably, given the stated intent of the two documents, *Changing Course* concentrates on the leadership role to be played by international corporations in promoting sustainable development. It devotes entire chapters to managing corporate change and pricing the environment, topics either ignored or not covered in depth in *Agenda 21*.

The Rio Declaration examines the role of states in protecting the environment during armed conflict and in settling disputes peacefully. It also underlines the important roles of women, youth and indigenous peoples in sustainable development. These groups do not receive special attention in *Changing Course*, which focuses on the special role of open and competitive markets in achieving a more environmentally secure future.

Summary

The greatest conformity on priorities and actions is between *Agenda 21* and *ASCEND 21* on issues related to the physical environment such as atmosphere and the marine environment. This is understandable, since members of ICSU served as scientific advisers for *Agenda 21*.

The agendas line up according to their primary commitments. Where making economic development is a priority, *Agenda 21* has more in common with *Changing Course* and the *Youth Action Guide* than with the other agendas, most of which dismiss increased prosperity or economic growth as a major goal.

The *NGO Alternative Treaties* address the greatest number of priority areas covered in *Agenda 21*. The treaties, however, emphasize issues such as alternative economic models and reduced military spending, and propose many actions that do not appear in *Agenda 21*. The language used in *Agenda Ya Wananchi* and *Voice of the Eagle* sets them apart from *Agenda 21*. These agendas rarely stray from spiritual and lifestyle issues and focus on the ethical or spiritual aspects of virtually every subject they discuss. The *Women's Action Agenda 21* stresses social environment issues over physical environment issues, while the reverse is true for *Agenda 21*. The *Global Assembly of Women and the Environment* gives prominence to good environmental management rather than development, while *Agenda 21* attempts to give both issues equal prominence. *Youth '92* focuses on the misdeeds of richer countries more forcefully than does *Agenda 21*.

A number of themes that recur in other agendas are either missing from *Agenda 21* or receive cursory treatment. These include ethical considerations, democracy, racism, alternative economic models, new definitions of development, regulation of transnational corporations, the urgent need to end all nuclear activities, and redirection of funds now used for military spending. The need to change personal attitudes and practices, while not completely missing from *Agenda 21*, gets much stronger coverage in *Caring for the Earth*, the *Youth Action Guide*, *Voice of the Eagle* and *Agenda Ya Wananchi*. Most agendas call for political activity such as lobbying or campaigning to achieve the stated objectives. This is not an important element of *Agenda 21*, *Changing Course* or *ASCEND 21*.

7

PROGRESS ON THE IMPLEMENTATION OF THE AGENDAS

The agendas under discussion here were aimed at various audiences. The primary recommendations were directed towards national governments but the agendas also contain suggestions for individuals, local governments, business managers, scientific researchers and NGO activists, among others.

The extent to which the intended users of the agendas have responded to their proposals varies widely. UNCED was the catalysing event for most of these documents and, five years later in June 1997, the United Nations General Assembly Special Session (UNGASS) on progress since the Earth Summit provided the occasion for a review of progress on a number of the agendas.

Updates on what has happened since the Earth Summit include the following:

- *Programme for the Further Implementation of Agenda 21* (adopted by the Special Session of the General Assembly, 23–27 June 1997);
- *The Way Forward: Beyond Agenda 21* (includes contributions from many of the organizers of the NGO *Alternative Treaties*);
- *NGO Report on the Convention to Combat Desertification*;
- *Local Government Implementation of Agenda 21*;
- *A Grassroots Reflection on Agenda 21* (co-ordinated by the Environment Liaison Centre International, a primary organizer of *Agenda Ya Wananchi*);
- *Report on the Implementation of the Agenda of Science for Environment and Development into the Twenty-first Century* (prepared by the same organization that co-ordinated *ASCEND 21*);
- *Five Years After Rio: Measuring Progress in the Implementation of the Convention on Biological Diversity* (prepared by IUCN, one of the main contributors to *Caring for the Earth*);
- *Lighting the Path to Progress: Women's Initiatives and an Assessment of Progress since the 1992 United Nations Conference on Environment and Development* (prepared by the Women's Environment and Development Organization, main organizers behind the *Women's Action Agenda 21*);
- *AIESEC's Learning from the New Concept of Development* (from the organization which wrote the *Youth Action Guide*);

- *Signals of Change: Business Progress towards Sustainable Development* (compiled by the World Business Council for Sustainable Development, principal author of *Changing Course*).

A year before UNGASS, the United Nations Department for Policy Co-ordination and Sustainable Development (DPCSD) began to encourage countries to prepare reports on their progress in implementing *Agenda 21*. DPCSD also summarized the past three years of national reports prepared for each Commission on Sustainable Development session since the Earth Summit and presented these to countries for review and reflection.

By the time delegates arrived at UNGASS, many countries had prepared comprehensive statements outlining the degree to which *Agenda 21* had been implemented. The document, which emerged from the Special Session – *Programme for the Further Implementation of Agenda 21* – contained the following statement among its opening paragraphs:

> We acknowledge that a number of positive results have been achieved, but we are deeply concerned that the overall trends for sustainable development are worse today than they were in 1992. We emphasise that the implementation of *Agenda 21* in a comprehensive manner remains vitally important and is more urgent now than ever.

Practical actions inspired by the agendas

The cause-and-effect relationship between agenda-setting and implementation of more sustainable practices is not always easy to isolate. As with any process, a number of factors make it difficult to establish a direct link between a certain action and the recommendations of an agenda. However, planning agencies will frequently cite an official document to justify their actions. As the following examples illustrate, there has been a great deal of activity designed to conform with recommendations for building a more sustainable world as outlined in the agendas that came into being around the time of UNCED.

Agenda 21

Agenda 21, often cited by local and national planners, international treaty negotiators and sustainable development activists, agreed to by representatives of governments and supported, to varying degrees, by national and international funding, has stimulated the most activity of all the sustainable development agendas presented here.

It has been pointed out that a large number of activities were a direct result of the UNCED process[52] such as:

- *Agenda 21*;
- *the Rio Declaration*;
- the Forestry Principles;
- *the Climate Change Convention*;
- *the Biodiversity Convention*;
- *the Desertification Convention*;
- the UN Commission on Sustainable Development (CSD);
- the CSD NGO/Major Groups Steering Committee to interface with the UN in the work of the CSD;
- the Conference on Small Island Developing States;
- the Conference on Straddling and Highly Migratory Fish Stocks;
- the Inter-governmental Panel on Forests;
- more than 2,000 *Local Agendas 21* around the world;
- more than 120 National Sustainable Development Councils;
- more than 120 National Sustainable Development strategies;
- the development of sustainable development indicators at the local and national level; and
- enhanced involvement of stakeholders in the UN, national and local decision-making process.

A number of the activities from this long list can be attributed more directly to *Agenda 21*, in particular the development of *Local Agendas 21* as spelled out in chapter 28, national sustainable development strategies (chapter 8) and the setting up of 'national co-ordination structures' for the follow-up of *Agenda 21* (chapter 37), interpreted by many countries as National Councils for Sustainable Development.

NGO Alternative Treaties

As discussed earlier in this chapter, the provisions of the *NGO Alternative Treaties* have not been widely implemented. However, there are some notable exceptions. One of the more durable and relevant NGO treaties appears to be the *NGO Alternative Treaty on Sustainable Agriculture*. This document has been kept alive primarily through the efforts of the World Sustainable Agriculture Association (WSAA). During Rio +5, a multi-stakeholder civil society event held in March 1997 to review progress since the Earth Summit, WSAA representatives stated that the *NGO Sustainable Agriculture Treaty*, a document developed during the Earth Summit by NGO and farmer representatives from around the world, went much further than *Agenda 21* in challenging the agricultural *status quo*. The *NGO Sustainable Agriculture Treaty* blames the global socio-economic and political system that promotes industrial agriculture in general, and so-called Green Revolution agriculture in particular, for the social and environmental crisis in agriculture. This kind of energy-intensive and chemical-dependent agriculture degrades the fertility of soils, intensifies the effect of droughts, pollutes water, increases salinity and compaction of soils, destroys genetic resources, wastes fossil fuel, contaminates food and contributes to climate change.

Many of the changes called for in the *NGO Treaty on Sustainable Agriculture* are being implemented in NGO- and farmer-initiated projects throughout the world.

ASCEND 21

The International Council of Scientific Unions conducted its own assessment of the implementation of *ASCEND 21* and reported the following results:

Strengthened cohesion and co-operation between scientific groups in different countries and across disciplines

ASCEND 21 brought the international scientific community together. With this came the realization that better results would be achieved by continuing to work together. The key is to create coalitions between teams of scientists so that data and methods can be shared and improved upon and duplication can be avoided, saving resources and time. Leadership and common policy are important, not only to save resources but also to strengthen the voice of science in reaching other communities. Enhanced communication technology has greatly helped this effort. Scientists can communicate by electronic mail and fax and much information is now available on the World Wide Web.

During the past few years, a number of new bodies have been set up within the ICSU framework to address issues raised at the ASCEND conference. Although established before the Earth Summit, ICSU's Advisory Committee on the Environment provides a cohesive base to co-ordinate ICSU's environmental activities.

Strengthening the capacities of developing countries is high on the agenda and various activities have been put in place to fulfil this. For example, ICSU members in Switzerland, Lebanon and Morocco have established joint initiatives and programmes to enhance North–South and South–South co-operation and partnership. ICSU has promoted co-operation through joint initiatives with the Third World Academy of Sciences (TWAS), the Earth Council and UNESCO, to address the problem of the isolation of scientists in developing countries. Core Programmes of Global Change projects provide many research and capacity-building opportunities. Other initiatives of science groups include special programmes to assist scientists in developing countries, such as workshops to reduce the gap between teaching and practice, research programmes, many teaching fellowship programmes, and student fellowships to enable participation in scientific meetings.

A growing network has emerged between national research councils and other bodies in different countries in a bid to improve international scientific relations and create a more united scientific community.

Enhanced communication and co-operation with decision-makers and
end-users of research

Communicating scientific results and assessments to decision-makers is an important part of the *ASCEND 21* recommendations and one which has been tackled during the past five years. There are now lists of programmes that are initiated by government and research institutes and funded by the private sector.

A growing trend in many countries is the creation of Ministries of the Environment, National Councils for the Environment and Committees on Environment and Development which, among other activities, promote co-operation between government ministries and NGOs. To compensate for diminishing national funds, these bodies also serve the purpose of increasing contact with international foundations and raising the country's research profile in the funding community.

Some Global Change research groups, such as the Finnish Research Programme on Climate Change, actively encourage interaction between their scientists and decision-makers. The group has sent questionnaires to expert organizations, government officials, politicians and NGO representatives. The results of the survey were compiled in a report and used as background material for a series of discussions.

Since Rio, many scientific bodies have increased their co-operation with intergovernmental organizations. This has allowed different audiences to be reached and increased the network of scientific knowledge. In this spirit, several Global Observing Systems are evolving their strategy to include governmental and non-governmental mechanisms.

International conventions have helped to mobilize public opinion and put pressure for change on the world's governments. The scientific community has been involved in the existing conventions on Ozone, Climate Change, Biodiversity and Desertification since their inception. The International Association on Water Quality (IAWQ) is proposing to implement *Agenda 21* recommendations in the area of freshwater by establishing a global Freshwater Convention, and several ICSU bodies already are working on the scientific aspects of water resources.

The consensus in the scientific community is that, with a growing number of links between those who make the decisions and the scientists who produce the data and assessments, there is a greater chance of the correct policy decisions being made.

Involvement of economics and the social sciences in global research
programmes

Another development since Rio is the establishment of interdisciplinary scientific programmes that include the social sciences and consider the economic and political aspects of global change. Ten years ago, the pure sciences would not have considered giving social sciences equal standing in problem analysis. *ASCEND 21* and UNCED promoted the need to include these areas when looking at global environmental problems.

The value of interdisciplinary research is enhanced by creating alliances between the natural, engineering, social and economic, human and medical sciences. The social and economic aspects of change cannot be ignored. A prime example of such a partnership is the establishment of an International Human Dimensions of Global Change Programme (IHDP) jointly sponsored by ICSU and the International Social Science Council (ISSC). Before 1996, this programme was supported only by the social science community. In its present form, it will bring together more natural and social scientists to begin looking at this important aspect of global change which has hitherto been neglected by the traditional 'hard' sciences.

SCOPE, ICSU's Scientific Committee on Problems of the Environment, which provides a mechanism and forum for producing credible assessments of environmental concerns, has also progressed to encompass economic and social science expertise. Projects such as Indicators of Sustainable Development illustrate how scientists can co-operate with governmental agencies from different countries and with intergovernmental agencies in order to develop instruments for sound decision-making for sustainable development. Another project on Groundwater Contamination produced several training seminars directed at decision-makers, engineers and technicians in liaison with the programme workshops.

Enhanced data accessibility

Data must be accessible if international co-operation and exchange of information are to be strengthened. Several chapters in *Agenda 21* point out the need for better collection and assessment of data. More and more scientific databases are being set up so that data can be shared by local and national planners and scientists around the world. ICSU has adopted several strong resolutions calling for the free and open access to scientific data and has been successful in preventing measures that threatened this access.

The advent of the World Wide Web has led to an explosion of data available to anyone possessing a computer, and the Internet has become a valuable tool for exchanging information. The Global Terrestrial Observing System (GTOS), for example, revised a Terrestrial Ecosystem Monitoring Sites Database (TEMS) developed by the United Nations Environment Programme (UNEP). This is available on the Web and is a useful compilation for anyone looking for appropriate terrestrial sites anywhere on Earth. The datasets provided by the IGBP Data and Information System on land surface, soils, biomass and terrestrial primary production are useful tools for decision-making.

Several capacity-building programmes promote the sharing of scientific research and environmental data through partnership with member countries in order to advance sustainable development of the region. The International Soil Reference and Information Centre (ISRIC) has developed the methodology for a World Soils and Terrain Digital Database which will be a valuable tool in setting priorities for global action and environmental assistance on soil and terrain conditions.

Women's Action Agenda 21

Many initiatives have resulted, at least in part, from the priorities identified in the *Women's Action Agenda 21*. These examples are drawn from the Women's Environment and Development Organization's report on *Women's Initiatives and an Assessment of Progress since the 1992 United Nations Conference on Environment and Development*. The examples, the report states, are 'by no means representative; rather [they] illustrate the complexities involved and the inspiration of what can be achieved'.

Giving women credit

Poor women face the greatest obstacles in borrowing money for a variety of legal, cultural and other reasons. Many NGOs around the world are currently engaged in delivering financial services to poor women, with high success and payback rates. Rural credit initiatives will become increasingly important to post-Rio implementation, especially as food production becomes less locally controlled and rural communities must search for alternative incomes.

NIGERIA

The Country Women Association of Nigeria (COWAN), led by Chief Bisi Ogunleye, a member of WEDO's board of directors and recipient of the 1996 Hunger Project Award, has administered an African Traditional Responsive Banking system since the early 1980s. Based on traditional savings and credit practices, the project now serves nearly 80,000 women throughout Nigeria. Borrowers typically use loans to expand food-processing activities – for example, cassava, palm oil, soybeans, maize and rice – or for small-scale manufacturing such as cloth, mats and pottery.

BANGLADESH

The Grameen Bank, both a bank and a poverty alleviation organization, was created after seven years of experimentation with an action research project intended to demonstrate that the poor can generate enough income from small enterprises to support small-scale lending. In 1983, Grameen became a government-lending bank to provide credit to the rural poor. Today, it is the largest operating NGO in Bangladesh, with more than 1,000 branches and 2 million members.

The Grameen Bank has also created great support for poor women. Women's participation in borrowing groups gives them the confidence and support to assert their rights to economic assets. Bangladeshi economist Mahbub Hossain, in interviews with 120 female borrowers, found evidence of increased social status of women. Women reported that husbands were more likely to treat them as equals. There was also less physical violence, threat of physical violence and verbal abuse.

Fighting unsustainable fishing practices

BANGLADESH

This is a particularly vivid example of how the Rio consensus is being undermined by global economic pressures, and to what lengths women must often go to resist and overcome destructive and dangerous practices.

Export shrimp cultivation in Bangladesh is fuelled by the drive for export earnings and demand from the North. People are prevented from growing food on land illegally occupied by shrimp farms and land near the farms is destroyed by salinity. Powerful shrimp farmers pay thugs and police to seize control over common lands, especially fragile mangrove ecosystems that are often the only resource to which poor families have access. Shrimp cultivation threatens the survival of large numbers of people as well as the mangroves of southwestern Bangladesh which are a vital nursery for fish and other sea life.

With support from prominent NGOs like Nijera Kori (Doing it Ourselves), landless people have mobilized against the shrimp farmers. As the primary targets of violence, men may be forced to go into hiding, leaving women to face police harassment. Some women have displayed remarkable bravery in confronting problems against which international agreements and institutions seem powerless. As one woman explained:

> My husband was in hiding for the last few days and I had no food in
> the house. On top of everything else, the police came into my home,
> used obscene language and pushed me around. I had no place to hide.
> I was pushed against the wall. I had no choice but to defend my chil-
> dren and myself with whatever I had. So I picked up my broom and
> beat the policeman with it.

In some areas, this type of resistance and activism has allowed people to keep their lands as shrimp-free zones, at least temporarily.

It is this sort of situation, however, which exposes the extent to which the Rio consensus can be rendered moot at the local level by international economic competition. As long as shrimp prices remain high and export earnings remain the highest priority, local food production will receive short shrift to the detriment of local people and ecosystems. Local involvement in the shrimp market may be viable and could be undertaken sustainably, but a major realignment of the shrimp industry would be necessary if its benefits were to become more universal.

The Women's Caucus: unprecedented power for women's advocacy at UN conferences

Since its inception, WEDO has facilitated the participation of NGO women through the Women's Caucus, held daily at five world conferences: UNCED, ICPD in Cairo, the Copenhagen Social Development Summit, the Beijing Women's Conference (where it was called the Women's Linkage Caucus) and Habitat II, held in Istanbul in June 1996. A Women's Caucus at the Human Rights Conference in Vienna was a vital force in the recognition that women's rights are human rights. Women also participated in a key negotiating session before the November 1996 World Food Summit in Rome to ensure that prior commitments made to women in Cairo and Beijing were reaffirmed in the final Food Summit documents.

Before this caucus process was launched at UNCED, the tendency in civil society might have been to dismiss the United Nations as a high-minded talk shop where words on paper carried no weight. Since UNCED, citizens, especially women, increasingly are holding governments accountable for taking international agreements seriously.

However, the constant need to protect past consensus from continued attempts by a handful of ideological interests to roll them back has cost vital time, money, energy and human resources that could have been better applied to advancing consensus on critical areas of implementation.

The objective of the Women's Caucus methodology, developed by WEDO and collaborating groups, is to mobilize women from every region around common agendas and to facilitate the participation of women from developing countries in policy advocacy.

Examining negotiating documents line by line, suggesting deletions and additions, women became skilled lobbyists, often working side by side with their national delegations in unprecedented peer acceptance. Success was sometimes achieved in a single critical word or paragraph. But, in the case of the ICPD documents, nearly two-thirds of the final recommendations of the Women's Caucus were reflected in the final Programme of Action.

Subsequent conferences, particularly the Copenhagen Social Development Summit and the Beijing Conference on Women, demonstrated that women are a powerful force in international negotiations. Largely as a result of the work of the Women's Caucus and many women's organizations, both the Copenhagen and Beijing conferences produced more concrete commitments by governments than had been expected during preparatory discussions.

Women's emergence as a force to be reckoned with at the UN is a major achievement since Rio. However, women continue to be disproportionately under-represented in senior positions within the UN administration and women heads of mission to the UN remain scarce. The task ahead is to translate the power women acquired in negotiating UN conference agreements to the institutions that oversee and control implementation.

Youth Action Guide

AIESEC has identified the following projects as good examples of how their organization understands sustainable development, based on the Brundtland Commission's *Our Common Future*, the *Youth Action Guide* and *Agenda 21*.

Student exchange to entrance sustainability

The purpose of the PRODESCO programme is to use the mechanism of student exchange to aid in the development of organizational and management structures for sustainability. This includes the creation of new income sources, training and environmental conservation in marginal sectors of Costa Rican society. It also involves fighting the negative effects of urbanization and promoting sustainable development through international and intersectoral understanding and co-operation. The project brings together more than thirty graduate or undergraduate students from different parts of the world and different backgrounds to develop a number of sustainable development projects and activities in communities with scarce resources.

AIESEC is not only seeking to provide a learning cultural experience for the trainees, but more importantly to apply their knowledge to the solution of certain needs of the communities involved with PRODESCO. What makes these communities special is that they include a number of families who are not only looking for better life conditions, but who are also willing to promote a number of social, environmental and sustainable values, and at the same time to build management structures that will ensure the continuity of the impact on and of the improvement in the community.

Building local sustainability

The PRODERE programme is the result of a partnership between UNDP, the Italian government and AIESEC to contribute to local sustainable development in areas inhabited by refugees from the Central American wars of the 1980s. The programme works using Agencies of Local Economic Development (ADEL) to co-ordinate existing resources or resources that come to the region from abroad.

The ADELs are run by community representatives, experts, technicians, and people seconded from UNDP, who co-ordinate their work with the students or recent graduates of AIESEC. The group's role consists of creating partnership opportunities between the entrepreneurial potential, working capability, the natural resources that can be used without harming ecosystems and the financial resources coming from external contributions. The agency does not pretend to be an economic planning institution, simply one of the actors that contributes to the development.

Students are selected from an international pool and spend between three and five months in the project. This provides an opportunity to expand cultural understanding of all the actors involved in local projects, contributing to the development of the community. The principal objective is to provide a realistic and concrete answer to the problem of under-development and marginalization through sustainable solutions in the medium and long term.

The underlying assumption is that economic development, no matter what indicators are used to measure it, is not an end in itself but must be understood as a means to improve the quality of life and to offer better opportunities to sectors of society's fringe-dwellers. In this way, economic development serves the larger goal of human development.

The project identifies the main problems that producers face every day. It stimulates the potential for community members to help themselves by providing access to the technical and financial resources needed to achieve the best solutions.

Changing Course

The World Business Council for Sustainable Development has reflected on the ways in which business has moved forward since the Earth Summit. *Changing Course* was the report that the WBCSD contributed to the Earth Summit process. The report itself is an example of a successful guide to planning for sustainability. It has been published in more than a dozen languages and is used as a basic text in many business schools around the world.[53]

The WBCSD identifies many initiatives arising out of *Changing Course* and the UNCED process, and points out that 'to some extent' business was already acting on some of these types of strategies before the Earth Summit.

Life-cycle analysis

Companies are increasingly using the developing science of life-cycle analysis (LCA), also called life-cycle assessment, to reduce the environmental impact of their products and production processes and to develop better products. In its crudest form, life-cycle analysis involves listing the various positive and negative environmental aspects of a specific product or process.

Xerox is using product life-cycle environmental assessment as a tool in its design-for-environment tool kit and has completed a streamlined life-cycle analysis of a small/mid-volume copier system. In this study Xerox views products and services as a system that serves office-document-processing needs. As an initial objective the company determines which aspect of its products and services contribute most significantly to the overall environmental impact of meeting these needs.

The results of the study indicate that paper manufacturing and energy use by the copier are the primary contributors to the machine's environmental impact throughout its life. These and other results are being used to support research and technology resource investment decisions and serve as a baseline to identify opportunities to improve environmental performance.

At Xerox, where managing by data and facts is fundamental, the LCA has provided the information necessary to quantify areas where the greatest improvements can be made. LCA can serve as a valuable tool in any company and acting on these opportunities can lead to substantial business benefits.

Xerox's experience shows that simple LCAs can provide value in research, technology, and design decision-making. But even for a large company, the value gained does not support the prohibitive expense of conducting comprehensive LCAs. Streamlined screening methodologies need to be developed and high-quality environmental inventory data for materials, process and parts need to be more readily accessible if LCAs are to be used widely.[54]

Screened investment funds

Screened, ethical or social funds exclude investments in the stocks of companies deemed to be unethical or environmentally irresponsible in favour of the stocks of other companies. The funds also strive to deliver competitive financial returns.

Findings of the Storebrand Scudder Environmental Value fund, so far, are that eco-efficient companies in general provide better returns on investment. During the fund's first six months, it outperformed the Morgan Stanley World International Capital Index (MSWICI) by 3 per cent and provided a net return to investors of nearly 9 per cent. It also outperformed Scudder's Global Themes Equity Fund, which is based on the same kind of fundamental financial analysis but without the eco-efficiency analytic screen.

A back-test of the fund's portfolio at launch showed that, if five years ago an investor had chosen to invest in the stocks the fund chose at launch, the investor would have received an average annual return of 22 per cent, which would have been nearly double the 12 per cent average annual return of the MSWICI.

It is too early to tell if the eco-efficiency analysis will consistently lead to superior investment performance in bull and bear markets, but results so far are promising and have generated a good deal of interest among investors and company environmental managers. Regulators in Sweden, Denmark, Germany and the United Kingdom are exploring how to strengthen environmental reporting standards in ways that will prove more useful to interested investors.

In short, the Storebrand Scudder Environmental Value Fund shows that environmental values can be integrated into investment management and that doing so results in significant benefits: first, capital flows to eco-efficient companies, thereby reducing their capital cost and financing their growth; second, investors do not sacrifice investment performance. They might even achieve superior financial returns.[55]

Social partnerships

Business traditionally has found it difficult to co-operate with its critics or follow the lead of organizations outside government. But the obvious change in corporate mood that followed Rio encouraged an unprecedented degree of exploration to find – through partnership – new solutions to some of the world's old environmental problems.

Fisheries that have sustained coastal communities for generations have declined rapidly in recent years. The United Nations Food and Agriculture Organization reports that seventy of the world's commercially important marine fish stocks are either fully fished, over-exploited, depleted or slowly recovering.

Unilever, the Anglo-Dutch corporation, and the World Wide Fund for Nature (WWF) have formed a conservation partnership to create market incentives for sustainable fishing by establishing an independent Marine Stewardship Council (MSC).

WWF and Unilever admit to different motives but shared objectives: to ensure the long-term viability of global fish populations and the health of the marine ecosystems on which they depend. Unilever, which has 20 per cent of the world frozen fish market, has committed itself to buying only certified fish by 2005. The MSC is looking for support from other organizations.

Unilever is committed to being responsive to the concerns of its consumers and wants to offer them the option to choose products from sustainable business practices. The MSC has the potential to affect significantly and positively the state of fisheries world-wide. The MSC will be shaped by an inclusive international consultation process engaging all stakeholders in the industry.

In tandem with this process, there is a ground-swell of international support for the MSC, encompassing industry, NGOs, politicians and others. These groups and individuals believe that the MSC has the potential to have a significant impact on the biological sustainability of fish stocks world-wide.

8

AGENDA-SETTING FOR
SUSTAINABILITY

It is clear from the preceding chapters that a great deal of effort went into drafting the agendas for environment and development that appeared around the time of UNCED. It is also apparent that there is much agreement on the severity of the problems that we are all facing. Yet five years later no national or local government, NGO, business or any other major player has been able to implement all the recommendations in any one of the agendas. The majority of the agendas discussed here have fallen by the wayside. *Agenda 21* stands alone as an agenda that still has relevance to many actors five years after it was drafted. But why is this the case?

To help answer this question it is useful to consider the agendas in four general categories:

- those put forward by non-governmental organizations that were politically active internationally (the *NGO Alternative Treaties*, *Agenda Ya Wananchi*, the *Women's Action Agenda 21*; the *Global Assembly of Women and the Environment*, *Youth '92*, *Voice of the Eagle* – an indigenous peoples' document rather than an NGO document);
- those originating from professional associations (*ASCEND 21*, *Changing Course*);
- those developed by established institutions (*Caring for the Earth*; the *Youth Action Guide on Sustainable Development*); and
- *Agenda 21*

The NGO documents

The agendas put forward by the international non-governmental organizations and networks suggested the greatest number of changes to the *status quo*. In most instances, they highlighted issues missing from *Agenda 21* such as alternative economic development models, regulation of transnational corporations, ending of nuclear activities and redirection of military spending towards supporting these types of changes. However, these agendas have all but disappeared. Even among those who were central to the drafting of the treaties they appear to have been forgotten. In *The Way Forward: Beyond Agenda 21*, a review of progress since the Earth Summit, a number of the contributors were very active in 1992 organizing the alternative-treaty process but there is no mention made of the treaties within that volume. The only agenda analysis in the book is aimed at the implementation of *Agenda 21*.

One of the co-ordinators of the treaty process has admitted that without an organized work-plan and serious commitment in each region of the world, it has not been possible to move from the drafting of text to implementation.[56] Another principal organizer from the Philippines, Patricia Araneta, has said, 'I believe that the content of the treaties and the process used in drawing them up have been very valuable parts of the whole process which made it possible for NGOs to have such a visible presence at the UN meetings.'

As illustrated in the previous chapters, there is more agreement than disagreement between *Agenda 21* and the *NGO Alternative Treaties*. The areas where they diverge generally reflect a fundamental difference in values, such as acceptance or rejection of the principles of unlimited economic growth. The inability of the NGOs involved in manufacturing the treaties to move them into action can be linked to broader issues of representativeness and accountability. These aspects of the NGO condition continue to plague NGOs as they struggle for recognition in international forums and to go beyond identifying problems to implementing solutions.

Agenda Ya Wananchi, more than the *NGO Alternative Treaties*, emerged from consultation with grassroots and community groups. Five years later one of the main co-ordinators of the agenda, the Environment Liaison Centre International based in Nairobi, released *A Grassroots Reflection on Agenda 21*. This document, like *The Way Forward*, made no mention of the agenda that they themselves had been so involved with during the time of the Earth Summit. The focus is, instead, on *Agenda 21*.

The *Women's Action Agenda 21*, the *Global Assembly of Women and the Environment* and *Youth '92* made it clear that one of their primary objectives in drafting an agenda was to highlight issues that might otherwise be overlooked in the government negotiations. As was mentioned earlier, the organized women's groups were seen as very successful in getting many of their recommendations relating to women into *Agenda 21*. This is less true for youth.

The contribution from a number of North American indigenous peoples, *Voice of the Eagle*, has very little similarity with *Agenda 21*. It remains a series of recommendations for attitudes that will bring about a more sustainable way of living. It is difficult to judge to what extent these suggestions have been accepted, although the lack of progress pointed out by the five-year review makes it seem unlikely that they have been widely recognized.

The evidence indicates that the agendas produced by different NGOs served primarily to broaden discussion in the governmental negotiations. This is no small feat, but it means that in areas where there were significant differences the NGO voice was not heard. As NGOs themselves are fond of pointing out, 'as much as people like to speak of the NGO community, there is no such thing'.[57] Indeed, the NGOs active on the international scene at the time of the Earth Summit were extremely diverse. Many of them were from an environmental background, having come into being during the Green Movement of the 1960s and early 1970s. The history of the Green Movement has been traced by Chatterjee and Finger, who indicate that this movement was 'fragmented' and 'taken by surprise by global ecology' by the time of UNCED. Development NGOs which were more familiar with trade and debt issues than with environmental concerns were active at UNCED, as were so-called special constituencies, including women, youth, farmers and fisherfolk, among others. There were scientists and academics and, where they did not meet with too much hostility, there was business and industry.

All of these different groups were keen to participate in the Earth Summit. They hoped to influence the text of the plan of action for UNCED. Some analysts feel strongly that by putting the emphasis on getting NGOs and other interested parties to be concerned about participation in UNCED the genuine underlying problems of the global crisis were overlooked. They believe that this situation continues to draw energies away from working towards real change: 'The obsession with establishing dialogue has diverted attention from the real issues, perpetuated business as usual, and contributed to co-opting and weakening the Green movement.'[58]

In retrospect, this assessment holds some validity when the fate of the *NGO Alternative Treaties* is acknowledged. It was no doubt helpful from a networking perspective for so many groups interested in change to meet together in one place, but what were the real changes brought about by the NGO activities relating to the Earth Summit? The Global Forum certainly allowed those working on the *NGO Alternative Treaties* to feel that they were accomplishing something. But it cannot have been a bad thing from the perspective of the official conference to have the majority of civil society activists letting off steam in a kind of parallel but not necessarily complementary process.

NGOs were also active in a number of the official delegations, and the nature of international negotiation makes it difficult to tease out their effect on the outcome of the Summit. However, this process is distinct from the NGO treaty-making that resulted in over forty agendas, signed by more than 3,000 people, that five years later are practically forgotten.

Professional associations

For the most part, the agendas that originated from professional organizations were in agreement with the objectives of *Agenda 21*. This is certainly true for much of *ASCEND 21*, compiled by the International Council of Scientific Unions (ICSU) who were the special advisers on science to the UNCED Secretariat. One of the principal authors of *Changing Course*, Stephan

Schmidheiny, was also a special adviser to Maurice Strong, the Secretary-General of UNCED.

These agendas were primarily directed at the members of the organizations that set them. An organized management structure supported by a skilled secretariat allowed both of these agendas to realize a certain level of implementation. The examples in Chapter 7 bolster this view.

Their agendas indicate that both ICSU and the World Business Council for Sustainable Development recognize the challenge presented by sustainability. Both appear to ascribe to problem-solving through an incremental approach without too much disruption to current models of development.

Established institutions

IUCN (a primary contributor to *Caring for the Earth*) and AIESEC (the authors of the *Youth Action Guide to Sustainable Development*) are organizations that have been in existence for decades. IUCN has a long history as an institution that brings together those interested in solving environmental problems and includes both NGOs and government agencies among its members. AIESEC, originally an organization for business students, has now broadened its membership and its mandate to include socio-economic and environmental projects among its programmes.

The agendas produced by these bodies are more specific in their recommendations than many of the other agendas. In the years following UNCED, both reorganized their structure based on their agendas and on *Agenda 21*. IUCN has been a leader in supporting the development and pushing for the implementation of the Convention on Biological Diversity. Biodiversity was an important theme in two of the chapters of *Caring for the Earth*. AIESEC has continued to focus on hands-on projects linking sustainability with community participation, a recurring theme throughout the *Youth Action Guide*.

Agenda 21

Nearly all of the review work done for the United Nations General Assembly Special Session five-year review on progress since Rio has focused on the implementation of *Agenda 21*. As mentioned above, even those who worked on their own agendas in 1992 had switched to reviewing progress in *Agenda 21* by 1997. *Agenda 21* is discussed in great detail in the previous chapters. A lot of planning and organizing has occurred in government agencies as a result of *Agenda 21* but the actual implementation of recommendations has been much more difficult to document.

There are a myriad reasons why we have not moved further on the implementation of *Agenda 21*. It is, indeed, easier to plan than to take action on any level, from the personal to the international. Vested interests resist change, aided by the complacency of some and the misfortune of others. This is certainly true among government agencies where it can take years for policies to move through the series of needed approvals.

There is also much risk and uncertainty surrounding sustainability. It is not clear that we know precisely what to do to avoid falling further into unsustainable practices. All the recommendations aside, a good number of strategies, such as alternative measurements for gross domestic product that evaluate economic growth using principles of sustainability, have not yet been tested on a large scale. In the area of the physical environment, fish stocks continue to decline in many parts of the globe, regardless of efforts to revive them.

Earth Summit Watch (ESW) has identified 'flaws in the decision-making model implicit in *Agenda 21*' as a major impediment to implementation. The model of decision-making and policy generation set out in *Agenda 21* 'is simply too expensive and complex to be achieved within ordinary societies'. ESW goes on to say that the implementation of *Agenda 21* relies on decision-making at the highest level, which is not always possible due to changing governments and that the methodology of integrating the different components of sustainability remains 'experimental'.

Lack of funding is another frequently cited culprit blocking the implementation of *Agenda 21*. It is a reality that there is not sufficient funding available but it is important to look at why this may be the case. In some countries resources are extremely scarce, and compliance with international agreements must be balanced with meeting the basic needs of the population. But in other instances, the unavailability of funding directly reflects the priorities of a nation. For many countries, developed and developing, economic growth remains the number one priority. This is at odds with all the NGO agendas discussed here but does not contradict either *Agenda 21* or *Changing Course*. It underlines a type of double vision among those working for sustainability, where there are those advocating real lifestyle and consumption changes for the rich and those who refuse to question current underlying conditions.

Another stumbling block to implementation, instantly recognizable to anyone working in the field of sustainable development, is competition among the major actors. Turf wars are rife throughout the sustainability movement. United Nations agencies compete for areas of influence and responsibility. NGOs battle it out for ideas and associated projects that may really make the difference. Research institutions fight to conduct investigations in parts of the world and on topics that are currently in vogue. It is one of the dirty secrets of the movement that organizations which frequently speak of the need for greater transparency are anything but transparent when it comes to their closest competitors.

An overall comparison of the agendas

A summary of the discussion in the previous chapters helps to highlight the fact that the objectives and recommendations in the agendas that deviate the least from the prevailing norms are the ones most likely to be implemented.

Similarities

As Table 8.1 illustrates, there are many shared fundamental principles and objectives across all the agendas. Out of the ten most frequently mentioned principles and objectives, nine are found in *Agenda 21*, the NGO *Alternative Treaties* and *Agenda Ya Wananchi*. Half are agreed to by *Agenda 21*, the NGO *Alternative Treaties*, *Agenda Ya Wananchi*, *Caring for the Earth* (four out of ten), *Youth '92* and *Changing Course*.

The objectives on which there is the greatest level of agreement relate to the social and economic environment and include putting an end to over-consumption and eliminating poverty. Many agendas link these issues and degradation of the physical environment. Even where these objectives are not clearly stated, the priorities and actions suggested indicate that they are important for all the agendas.

Principles guiding environment and development activities for which there is broad agreement include considering the needs of future generations, adopting the 'precautionary principle' (that is, erring on the side of caution when the effect on the environment is unknown), increasing participation in decision-making, respecting the knowledge of indigenous peoples and co-operating internationally to achieve a more sustainable existence.

Priorities

No single issue is given priority treatment by all the agendas considered here and, as was pointed out in Chapter 2, many of the topics raised are complex and interconnected. Every agenda illustrates a somewhat different understanding of the environment and development issues that currently require thought and action.

Education, including increasing awareness of environment and development issues, is addressed in nine out of the eleven agendas. Biodiversity, technology and water resources are brought to the fore in eight, while agriculture, atmosphere, population, trade and debt are highlighted in seven. Biotechnology, poverty and deforestation are given primary focus in over half of the agendas. Other subjects are raised as priorities in less than half of the agendas.

Obviously, it is not only the number of times that a topic is identified as a priority issue that is important but also the level of agreement regarding proposed actions. The greatest consensus surrounds activities for eliminating or controlling observable degradation of air, land or water, including direct impacts such as air or water pollution or indirect impacts such as effects on human health. Even in these areas where agreement exists, there is little measurable progress.

Table 8.1 Shared principles and objectives for environment and development

	Rio Declaration on Environment and Development (AGENDA 21)	NGO Alternative Treaties	Agenda Ya Wananchi	Ascend 21*	Caring for the Earth	Women's Action Agenda 21	Global Assembly of Women*	Youth '92	Youth Action Guide	Voice of the Eagle	Changing Course
Eliminate over-consumption	✓	✓	✓		✓	✓		✓			✓
Alleviate poverty	✓	✓	✓		✓	✓		✓			✓
The North should accept greater responsibility for current problems	✓	✓	✓					✓			
Greater participation in decision-making	✓	✓	✓			✓		✓			✓
Increase participation of women in decision-making	✓	✓	✓				✓	✓†			
International co-operation is needed to achieve sustainable development	✓		✓						✓†		✓
Adopt the precautionary principle	✓	✓	✓								✓
Respect the knowledge of indigenous peoples	✓	✓	✓		✓✓					✓	✓
Consider the needs of future generations	✓	✓	✓		✓			✓		✓	✓
Decrease disparities in standards of living	✓	✓	✓			✓					✓

*These agendas were presented in a manner that did not allow for the identification of specific principles and objectives aside from the reason for writing the agenda.

†Global partnership of youth

Identifying the actors who will make a difference

One of the main differences in the agendas' stated objectives and principles concerns the level at which action on environment and development problems should take place. The agendas all recognize that national governments have a role to play, but *Agenda 21*, being an agreement among governments, focuses most closely on the responsibility of governments. *ASCEND 21*, although it came into being primarily to clarify the position of the scientific community within the context of integrating environment and development, is also directed at policy- and decision-makers at the national, regional and local levels. *Changing Course* places a fairly heavy emphasis on 'working with governments' on a number of issues as well as encouraging actions within the business and industrial community. *Agenda Ya Wananchi* divides its action plan between appeals to governments and commitments by citizens' organizations.

The remainder of the agendas – *Caring for the Earth*, the *NGO Alternative Treaties*, the *Women's Action Agenda 21*, the *Global Assembly of Women and the Environment*, *Youth '92*, the *Youth Action Guide* and *Voice of the Eagle* – stress the need for personal commitment to lifestyle changes and for participation and innovation at the community and local levels. The five-year review has indicated that governments have taken action primarily in planning for implementations rather than implementation itself. It is not clear whether this is due to lack of time – five years is not really that long – or results from a lack of commitment. Organizations such as IUCN, WEDO, WBCSD and AIESEC remain actively attempting to realize sustainability in their areas of influence.

Who or what is responsible for current problems?

For some of the agendas, the need to place the blame for existing environment and development problems is an important theme. Among several of the agendas – namely, *Agenda 21*, the *NGO Alternative Treaties*, *Agenda Ya Wananchi* and *Youth '92* – there is agreement that richer, more developed countries (often referred to as 'the North') bear a responsibility for global conditions such as atmospheric pollution, contamination of the oceans and widespread poverty which far exceeds their share of the world's population. The remaining agendas do not place such emphasis on the undesirable behaviour of the richer countries but concentrate on problems arising from a lack of spiritual or moral focus (the *Women's Action Agenda 21*, *Voice of the Eagle*) or on development which strays from ecological principles, such as recognizing and protecting cultural and biological diversity (*Agenda Ya Wananchi*) or recognizing the limits to the Earth's carrying capacity (*Caring for the Earth*).

Degree of change required

All of the agendas address the need for change based on existing and ongoing environmental degradation and past approaches to development which have been largely unsuccessful. While some agendas, particularly *Agenda 21*, *ASCEND 21* and *Changing Course*, are critical of the current state of the environment and world development, they accept that existing institutions can be useful in resolving or reducing problems. Many of the agendas insist on the implementation of international agreements such as the *United Nations Convention on the Law of the Sea*, the *United Nations Declaration on Human Rights* or the *Montreal Protocol on Ozone*. But for other agendas, just improving the current system is not enough. They call for a complete rejection of the existing 'international model of development [which] results in social inequality and degradation of the environment' (*NGO Alternative Treaties*).

The greatest barriers to achieving sustainability may be rooted in this area of debate. The UNGASS review has indicated little progress since Rio. Fundamental assumptions underlying the prevailing economic system and its causal link to social development and sustainable ecosystems could be impeding any real change.

While *Agenda 21* acknowledges the imbalance between developed and developing regions it does not advocate changes in the form or structure of the international marketplace or any specific wealth redistribution schemes. Suggestions of this nature are found in agendas like the *Women's Action Agenda 21* and many of the *NGO Alternative Treaties*. In *Agenda 21*, *Changing Course* and *ASCEND 21* there is no systematic evaluation of the context in which sustainable practices persist. If we cannot openly recognize the reasons for blockages in the system which delivers sustainability, an effective response seems improbable at best.

Use of the term 'sustainable development'

Although sustainable development is a stated objective for a number of agendas, there is no agreement on the definition of this term. Some agendas use it without explaining its meaning. Others, such as *Changing Course* or the *Youth Action Guide*, use the definition offered by the Brundtland Commission; that is, that sustainable development means 'development that meets the needs of the present without compromising the ability of future generations to meet their own needs'. A number of agendas reject the term. 'The world community talks of sustainable development as the only strategy to conserve the limited natural resources of this troubled planet,' says *Voice of the Eagle*. 'Indigenous People are mainly interested in developing sustainability and protecting our sustainable traditional way of life.' *Agenda Ya Wananchi* says:

A different way of development is necessary, one which is sustainable and where ecological and social concerns for all humanity and future generations are given priority. However such sustainable development is incompatible with quantitative growth. Therefore the concept of sustainable development, as seen by the Brundtland report, is inherently contradictory.

Caring for the Earth characterizes sustainable development as being different from sustainable growth, and sees the two terms as contradicting each other. It defines sustainable development as 'improving the quality of human life while living within the carrying capacity of supporting ecosystems'. Five years after the drafting of these agendas consultations were carried out with National Councils for Sustainable Development (or similar bodies) in more than sixty countries. The results indicated that 'an operational definition of sustainable development' was a pressing need.[59]

Economic principles

Basing the concept of development on certain economic principles is seen as desirable in some agendas but not in others. *Agenda 21*, *Changing Course* and the *Youth Action Guide* see the benefits of trade liberalization and economic structural adjustment programmes in resolving environment and development problems. Other agendas suggest that the choice of economic solutions reflects a certain set of values, including a positive correlation between increased material wealth and quality of life. This line of reasoning is rejected by the *Women's Action Agenda 21*, *Agenda Ya Wananchi*, *Voice of the Eagle* and *Youth '92*.

Conclusions

There is more agreement than disagreement among the agendas, particularly on questions relating to the physical environment, including freshwater, the atmosphere, deforestation and the oceans. Here people are able to see evidence of damage or degradation. The scientific community can identify such evidence and pose responses which will control or eliminate problems, particularly small-scale or local ones.

Issues relating more directly to the human environment, including biotechnology, capacity building, consumption patterns, military considerations, population, poverty and waste, are addressed in a less uniform manner throughout the agendas although the majority of priorities and objectives raised are not contradictory.

The major differences among the agendas are found in the broader realm of who to blame for environment and development problems. There is a distinction between those who feel that the entire current approach to development and its interaction with the environment is seriously flawed and must be rejected, and those who indicate that, while there are problems with the present way of doing things, the system requires repair rather than replacement. The most dramatic example of this is in economics, where trade, debt, market mechanisms and income and lifestyle disparities between rich and poor are hotly contested across the agendas. This was so in 1992, and the 1997 UNGASS review indicated that sustainability remains elusive for many of these issues.

The fundamental difference among these documents is the ethical framework for problem definition, priority determination and potential actions. There is no basic shared belief among the agendas as to what constitutes right and wrong. More specifically, what is the correct definition of development? What is fair trade? Does the North have a moral obligation to the South based on past wrong? These questions remain as unresolved in 1997 as they did five years earlier.

The agendas apportion a lot of blame based on differing interpretations of the problems. The more commonly cited wrongdoers are national governments and business and industry, especially transnational corporations, and in many cases governments and large-scale industry do bear a heavy responsibility for existing problems. But, as a number of the agendas stress, much of this could be rectified through change on a personal level, including clarification of personal values and individual commitment to a more sustainable lifestyle.

The official UN review of progress since the Earth Summit did not identify a great deal of advance on anyone's definition of the sustainable development agenda. Many of the other agendas published at the time of UNCED have disappeared. The World Business Council for Sustainable Development is one of the few organizations that take a positive view of progress on sustainability.

As the previous chapters show, agenda-setting can be linked to a number of changes that engender sustainability. It is not necessarily the recommendations made in various agendas that precipitate action but rather the agenda-setting process itself. This process focuses on identifying problems, proposed solutions and those responsible for carrying out suggested actions.

In the final analysis, the agendas where it is clear that a number of recommendations have been turned into action are those that have an organized institutional or management structure supporting implementation. This includes the government agreement *Agenda 21*, the International Council of Scientific Union's *ASCEND 21*, the section on biodiversity in *Caring for the Earth*, AIESEC's *Youth Action Guide* and the World Business Council on Sustainable Development's *Changing Course*.

The *NGO Alternative Treaties*, spearheaded by the International NGO Forum, *Agenda Ya Wananchi*, co-ordinated by the Environment Liaision Centre International, *Youth '92* and *Voice of the Eagle* were more important as documents that presented alternative views about current paths.

Many people have worked hard in the past, and continue to do so today, to find a way to move ahead on sustainability. The very existence of the agendas illustrates that there are many individuals and groups who are unwilling to accept that the obstacles to problem-solving are insurmountable, thus justifying the title of this book.

The experience of setting agendas for achieving sustainable development has taught us that there is common ground among various interest groups. Even where a number of differences arise, cultural and biological diversity may dictate that a multiplicity of approaches is necessary. There might not only be one way of doing things. On the other hand, there are real differences in the belief systems that are motivating people to work for sustainability. In some cases, particularly in the area of economics, opposing views are at the heart of what is blocking genuine change.

The UNCED experience of agenda-setting has also demonstrated that for all the criticism directed at national governments, they are still perceived as the most powerful instruments for implementing sustainability. *Agenda 21*, essentially an agreement among nation states, continues to define sustainability for most of the major actors.

The problems we are facing have not diminished. Moving forward will require the courage to expose the differences among us which are impeding sustainability and the creativity to design strategies for getting past them. Perhaps it was shared hope for a better world that prompted the drafting of all the agendas, and perhaps it is exactly that which will propel us to a better, more sustainable future.

NOTES

1 A BIG BUILD-UP

1 Rachel Carson (1962) *Silent Spring*, New York: Houghton Mifflin Company.
2 John McCormick (1989) *The Environmental Movement: Reclaiming Paradise*, London: Belhaven Press.
3 Michael Grubb, Matthias Koch, Abby Munson, Francis Sullivan and Koy Thomson (1993) *The 'Earth Summit' Agreements: A Guide and Assessment*, Energy and Environment Programme, London: The Royal Institute of International Affairs/Earthscan Publications.
4 Commission on Global Governance (1995) *Our Global Neighbourhood*, Oxford: Oxford University Press.
5 World Commission on Environment and Development (1987) *Our Common Future*, Oxford: Oxford University Press.
6 United Nations Conference on Environment and Development (1992) *Report of the United Nations Conference on Environment and Development*, Rio de Janeiro: chapter 1, annex II.
7 Quoted in *The Earth Times*, 23 June 1997 'Review of Rio Earth Summit draws world leaders but doubts persist on commitment'.
8 *Programme for the Further Implementation of Agenda 21*, adopted by the Special Session of the General Assembly, 23–27 June 1997.
9 *Alternative Treaties* (1992) International NGO Forum, Philippine Secretariat and Philippine Institute of Alternative Futures, Manila.
10 *Agenda Ya Wananchi: Citizens' Action Plan for the 1990s* (1992) Nairobi: Environment Liaison Centre International (ELCI).
11 J.C.I. Dooge, G.T. Goodman, J.W.M. la Riviere, J. Marton-Lefevre, T. O'Riordan and F. Praderie (1992) *An Agenda of Science for Environment and Development into the Twenty-first Century*, Cambridge: Cambridge University Press.
12 IUCN/UNEP/WWF (1991) *Caring for the Earth: A Strategy for Sustainable Living*, Gland, Switzerland.
13 *Official Report: World Women's Congress for a Healthy Planet* (1992) Women's Environment and Development Organization (WEDO), New York.
14 Senior Women's Advisory Group on Sustainable Development of the United Nations Environment Programme (1992) *Global Assembly of Women and the Environment, 'Partners in Life': Final Report*, Washington, DC: UNEP.
15 *Youth '92: The World Youth Statement and Plan of Action on Environment and Development* (1992) Youth '92 Secretariat/Comisión Preparatoria Costarricense Juventud 92, Ottawa/Guadalupe.
16 *Youth Action Guide on Sustainable Development* (1991) Brussels: AIESEC International.
17 Alvin Manitopyes and Dave Courchene, Jr (1992) *Voice of the Eagle*, Calgary: Calgary Aboriginal Awareness Society.

18 Stephan Schmidheiny with Business Council for Sustainable Development (1992) *Changing Course: A Global Business Perspective on Development and the Environment*, Cambridge, MA: Massachusetts Institute of Technology.

2 THE AGENDA-SETTING PROCESS

19 Maximo T. Kalaw, Jr (1992) 'The NGO Treaties: from active resistance to creative alternative making', in *Alternative Treaties*, International NGO Forum, Philippine Secretariat and Philippine Institute of Alternative Futures, Manila.
20 IUCN/UNEP/WWF (1991) *World Conservation Strategy: Living Resource Conservation for Sustainable Development*, International Union for the Conservation of Nature and Natural Resources.
21 IUCN/UNEP/WWF (1991) op. cit.
22 Women are not specifically mentioned in chapter 2 (International Co-operation to Accelerate Sustainable Development in Developing Countries and Related Domestic Policies), chapter 9 (Atmosphere), chapter 16 (Biotechnology), chapter 22 (Radioactive Wastes), chapter 27 (Role of NGOs), chapter 37 (International Co-operation for Capacity Building) and chapter 39 (International Legal Instruments).

3 ECONOMIC CONSIDERATIONS

23 United Nations Department for Policy Co-ordination and Sustainable Development (1997) *Programme for the Further Implementation of Agenda 21*. Adopted by the Special Session of the General Assembly, 23–27 June 1997, New York.
24 Bjorn Stigson (1997) The Business Charter for Sustainable Development, in *The Way Forward: Beyond Agenda 21*, London: Earthscan.
25 Peter Padbury (1997) The NGO View of the Next Ten Years: Thoughts on Moving from the Basement of the UN to Global Implementation, in *The Way Forward: Beyond Agenda 21*, London: Earthscan.
26 Women's Environment and Development Organization (1997) *Lighting the Path to Progress*, New York: The Women's Environment and Development Organization.
27 Lester R. Brown, Michael Renner and Christopher Flavin (1997) *Vital Signs 1997* New York: W.W. Norton & Company.
28 Bangladesh Centre for Advanced Studies (1997) *Poverty, Environment and Sustainable Development*, Dhaka: Bangladesh Centre for Advanced Studies.
29 Charles Arden-Clarke (1997) *Trade Globalisation and Sustainable Development*, Gland: Earth Council/World Wildlife Fund.
30 Konrad Moltke (1997) *Trade and Sustainable Development*, Winnipeg: International Institute for Sustainable Development.

4 SOCIAL DEVELOPMENT

31 Carol Zinn (1997) *Special Focus Report on Education: Project Global 2000*, New York: Earth Council/Global Education Associates.
32 International Research Institutes (1997) *Public Perceptions of Environment/Health Link*, Toronto: IRI.
33 Rosalie Bertell (1997) *Health and the Environment*, Toronto: International Institute for Public Health.
34 Chip Linder (1997) *Agenda 21*, in *The Way Forward: Beyond Agenda 21*, London: Earthscan.
35 Ibid.
36 International Council for Local Environmental Initiatives (1997) *Local Government Implementation of Agenda 21*, Toronto: ICLEI.

37 Pratap Chatterjee and Matthias Finger (1994) *The Earth Brokers: Power, Politics and World Development*, London: Routledge.
38 Felix Dodds (ed.) (1997) *The Way Forward: Beyond Agenda 21*, London: Earthscan.
39 Lester R. Brown, Michael Renner and Christopher Flavin (1997) *Vital Signs*, New York: W.W. Norton & Company.
40 Women's Environment and Development Organization (1997) *Lighting the Path to Progress: Women's Initiatives and an Assessment of Progress since the 1992 United Nations Conference on Environment and Development (UNCED)*, New York: Women's Environment and Development Organization.

5 THE WELL-BEING OF ECOSYSTEMS

41 Gerardo Budowski (1977) *Ecosystems Management as a Tool for Sustainable Development*, Costa Rica: Earth Council/University for Peace.
42 Climate Network Europe (1977) *Climate Politics in Western Europe: Regional and Global Dimensions*, Brussels: Climate Network Europe.
43 For agendas which treat biodiversity and biotechnology separately, see 'Biotechnology', which follows this section.
44 World Conservation Union (1997) *Five Years after Rio: Measuring Progress in the Implementation of the Convention on Biological Diversity*, Gland: IUCN.
45 Carole Saint-Laurent (1977) 'The Forest Principles and the Intergovernmental Panel on Forests', in *The Way Forward: Beyond Agenda 21*, London: Earthscan.
46 Ibid.
47 Richard Ledgar (1997) *NGO Report on the Convention to Combat Desertification* (RIOD) Adelaide: The International NGO Network on Desertification and Drought.
48 Christopher Flavin (1977) *The Power to Choose – Creating a Sustainable Energy Future*, Washington, DC: Worldwatch Institute
49 Energy 21 (1997) *Energy for a Sustainable Tomorrow*, Paris: Earth Council/Energy 21.
50 Helene Connor (1997) *Is Energy Currently Contributing to Sustainable Development?* Paris: Earth Council/Global Energy Observatory.
51 Elizabeth Mann Borgese (1997) *Sustainable Development in the Oceans*, Halifax: International Oceans Institute.

7 PROGRESS ON THE IMPLEMENTATION OF THE AGENDAS

52 Jonathon Porritt (1979) Introduction to *The Way Forward: Beyond Agenda 21*, London: Earthscan Publications.
53 Stephan Schmidheiny, Rodney Chase and Livio De Simone (1997) *Signals of Change: Business Progress towards Sustainable Development*, Geneva: The World Business Council for Sustainable Development.
54 Contributed by Paul A. Allaire, Chairman and Chief Executive Officer, Xerox Corporation.
55 Contributed by Age Korsvold, President and Chief Executive Officer, Storebrand.

8 AGENDA-SETTING FOR SUSTAINABILITY

56 Patricia Araneta, personal communication, August 1977.
57 Peter Mucke (1997) 'Non-governmental organizations', in *The Way Forward: Beyond Agenda 21*, London: Earthscan.
58 Pratap Chatterjee and Matthias Finger (1994) *The Earth Brokers: Power, Politics and World Development*, London: Routledge:
59 Earth Council (1997) *Implementing Sustainability: Experiences and Recommendations from National and Regional Consultations for the Rio +5 Forum*, San José, Costa Rica: Earth Council.

INDEX

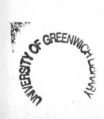